Manipal Manual of
PHYSIOLOGY

for

**Nursing • Allied Health Sciences • Pharmacy •
Alternative Systems of Medicine • MBBS • Dentistry**

Manipal Manual of
PHYSIOLOGY

for

Nursing • Allied Health Sciences • Pharmacy • Alternative Systems of Medicine • MBBS • Dentistry

C.N.Chandra Shekar Ph.D.

Dept. of Physiology,
Kasturba Medical College,
MANIPAL – 576 104, INDIA.

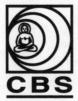

CBS PUBLISHERS & DISTRIBUTORS

NEW DELHI • BANGALORE   (INDIA)

Dedicated to

To my beloved mother late Smt. Shivamma C.N.

My alma mater, Kasturba Medical College,
A Constituent College of
Manipal Academy of Higher Education

My beloved teachers and students

ISBN : 81-239-1285-4

First Edition : 2006

Publishing Director : Vinod K. Jain

Published by :
Satish Kumar Jain for CBS Publishers & Distributors,
4596/1-A, 11 Darya Ganj, New Delhi - 110 002 (India)
E-mail: cbspubs@vsnl.com • Website: www.cbspd.com

Branch Office :
2975, 17th Cross, K.R. Road, Bansankari 2nd Stage, Bangalore-70
Fax : 080-26771680 • E-mail : cbsbng@vsnl.net

Printed at :
Swastik Packagings, Delhi-110 092

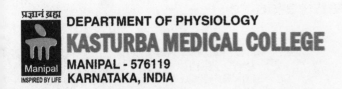 **DEPARTMENT OF PHYSIOLOGY**
KASTURBA MEDICAL COLLEGE
MANIPAL - 576119
KARNATAKA, INDIA

Phone: 08252 571201
      Ext. 22321, 22536
Fax: 08252 570500, 570062
Telex: 833-231 MAHE IN
E-mail: physiology@kmc.manipal.edu

Foreword

I am glad that Dr. C.N. Chandrashekar, Associate Professor of Physiology, has brought out a short manual of Physiology for students of Allied Health professional courses especially for dental students. Dr. Chandrashekar is eminently suited to write such a textbook.

He has been adjudged as one of the 'Good Teachers' in the College of Dental Surgery in 1993. In 2002 and 2004, he has been adjudged as one of the 'Good Teachers' in Kasturba Medical College, Manipal. The short manual he has written covers areas in which questions are asked in written and oral examinations. I am sure not only students of Allied Health Sciences but also students of I.MBBS will find it very helpful to revise quickly the whole subject.

May 23, 2005

Dr. A. Krishna Rao
Emeritus Professor,
Department of Physiology,
Kasturba Medical College, Manipal

Preface

Teaching the students of heterogeneous courses in health sciences in the last almost a quarter century made me realize that most of the books available in physiology have been designed to cater to the needs of the medical students only. Even here when the duration of the pre-clinical curriculum of medical graduate students has got reduced to barely nine months as against the erstwhile period of fourteen months or so, to gather all information in a succinct form is very difficult. Hence it was felt that presentation of concepts and facts in an unadorned form is very much warranted.

With the aforesaid aims and objectives, it was envisaged to present physiology of human body in the form of a manual that can accomplish the needs of health science graduate students in general. Efforts have been made to present the material in a much simplified and easily readable way. In many of the places flowcharts have been incorporated for better understanding and reproducibility. Some of the pertinent aspects, which a student cannot compromise upon, have been given in boxes. At most of the places the diagrams have been given in colour for better presentation and differentiation.

Hope this sincere attempt will be able to fulfill the long-standing aspirations of the students to get many of the pressing information from a single source and which can be referred to easily even at short notice period when one is in the midst of the examinations. I do wish and hope the students would definitely get benefited from this endeavour.

Constructive criticisms from all the quarters are expressly solicited. Wish you all the best.

C.N. Chandra Shekar
Deptt. of Physiology,
Kasturba Medical College,
Manipal – 576 104 (India)

Acknowledgment

While preparing this manual a number of people have helped, cooperated and guided me. It is my privilege and honour to express gratitude for the same.

- First and foremost thanks to Dr. A. Krishna Rao, former dean and professor emeritus of the department and a guiding spirit to most of us in the department. He has been a teacher par excellence for more than fifty years. I immensely thank him for going through the draft and also writing foreword for the book.

- Ever since the conception of thought of writing this manual, Dr. P. Laxminarayan Rao, another former dean and professor in the department, took time off even at short notices to go through the manuscript. He gave many esteemed suggestions for better presentation of the material. I am grateful to him for the same.

- I would like to thank my professor and head of my department Dr. Susan Benjamin for all the cooperation extended to me.

- My colleagues in the department Ms. Archana and Dr. Rajshree Ravishankar also helped me in checking the manuscript and preparation of the index. Indeed I sincerely acknowledge their help. I would also like to acknowledge and thank the help rendered by Mr. Santhosh of our department.

- A colleague and friend of mine who was after me all the time to bring out this manual is Dr. Rajgopal Shenoy, professor of surgery of our college. He constantly coaxed me to complete the task. I immensely thank him for the same.

- Without the able computer assistance, the manual would not have got completed in due period. I profusely thank Mr. Lobo Wilfred of M/s Chetana Communications, Mangalore for the same.

- I take this opportunity to thank Mr. S.K. Jain, Mr. V.K. Jain, Directors of M/s CBS Publishers & Distributors, New Delhi and to Mr. B.R. Sharma of the same organization for having agreed to publish the manual.

- My spouse Ms. Nandini Shekar and children Shashank Shekar and Shubhank Shekar for sparing me to complete this task duly deserve last but not the least thanks.

C.N. Chandra Shekar

Contents

Contents

Blood

CHAPTER 1

INTRODUCTION

Study of blood and its components is known as hematology. Blood is homogenous fluid connective tissue, which is in constant circulation throughout the body. In a normal person weighing 70 kg the volume of blood will be about 5 litres or in relation to body weight it will be about 70 ml/kg.

As specified earlier blood is homogenous connective tissue. *Broadly speaking it is composed*

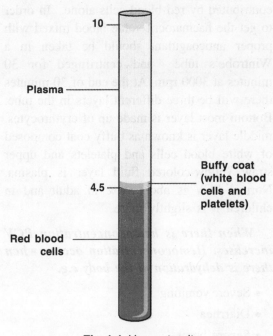

Fig 1.1 Haematocrit

Labels in figure:
- 10
- Plasma
- Buffy coat (white blood cells and platelets)
- 4.5
- Red blood cells

of two distinct parts namely a) plasma and b) formed elements. In terms of percentage, plasma constitutes 55% and the rest by the formed elements 45% (Fig. 1.1). Among the formed elements there are red blood cells, white blood cells and platelets. Major part of the formed element is contributed by the red blood cells. And the haematocrit or PCV (packed cell volume) value is normally given as 45%.

Plasma

All the formed elements of blood are in the suspended state in plasma. Plasma is made up 91-93% of water and organic and inorganic constituents form the remaining percentage.

Haematocrit (PCV - Packed cell volume - Fig. 1.1)

It is the percentage volume of blood that is contributed by red blood cells alone. In order to get the haematocrit value blood mixed with proper anticoagulant should be taken in a Wintrobe's tube and centrifuged for 30 minutes at 3000 rpm. At the end of 30 minutes there will be three different layers in the tube. Bottom most layer is made up of erythrocytes, middle layer is known as buffy coat composed of white blood cells and platelets and upper straw yellow-colored fluid layer is plasma. Normal PCV is about 45% in adult and in children it is slightly more.

When there is hemoconcentration PCV increases. Hemoconcentration occurs when there is dehydration of the body e.g.

- Severe vomiting
- Diarrhea
- Severe burns

In hemodilution PCV decreases e.g.

- Severe anemias

Functions of blood

- **Respiratory function:** Transport of oxygen to the tissues from lungs and carbon dioxide from tissues to the lungs.

- **Excretory function:** Carrying of metabolic wastes like urea, uric acid and creatinine to the kidney for excretion from the body.

- **Nutritive function:** Supply of the absorbed nutritive substances from the alimentary tract to almost all the parts of body.

- **Regulation of body temperature:** Help in the thermal balance of the body by contributing for the various physical and physiological mechanisms of heat transfer along the thermal gradient.

- **Protective function:** With the help of leucocytes and antibodies present in plasma, blood helps the body to sustain resistance against infections.

Specific gravity is the relative density of blood to that of water. The specific gravity of blood and its components is as follows:

Whole blood is about	1055 – 1060
Plasma alone	1025 – 1030
Formed elements only	1085 – 1090

PLASMA

As stated earlier apart from water, the other substances present in plasma are organic and inorganic in nature.

Some of the important organic substances are

- *Plasma proteins*
- *Urea*
- *Uric acid*
- *Creatinine*
- *Glucose*
- *Free fatty acids.*

Inorganic substances are

- *Sodium*
- *Potassium*
- *Calcium*
- *Iron*
- *Chloride.*

Plasma proteins: Total plasma protein concentration is about 6-8 g%. The concentration of different types of plasma proteins will be

- Albumin 4 – 5 g%, Molecular weight 68000.
- Globulin 2.3 g%, molecular weight varies from 90000 to 1300000. The different fractions are alpha 1 & 2, beta 1 & 2 and gamma globulins.
- Prothrombin 15 – 40 mg%
- Fibrinogen 0.3 g %, Molecular weight 330000.

Normal albumin globulin ratio is 2:1. Most of the plasma proteins are synthesized in liver ex-

cept gamma globulins, which are produced in the lymphoid tissue.

Separation of plasma proteins can be done by various techniques like:

- **Electrophoresis**
- **Immunoelectrophoresis**

Functions of plasma proteins

1. **Maintenance of colloidal osmotic pressure** which is about 25 mm Hg. Albumin contributes for 80% of colloidal osmotic pressure because the concentration of this protein is more in plasma. The maintenance of this pressure is essential to regulate the fluid volume in the intravascular compartment and interstitial spaces. In case this pressure decreases it can lead to accumulation of excess of fluid in the tissue spaces causing edema. Normally edema is seen in severe liver disorders, loss of plasma proteins in urine and in malnutrition.

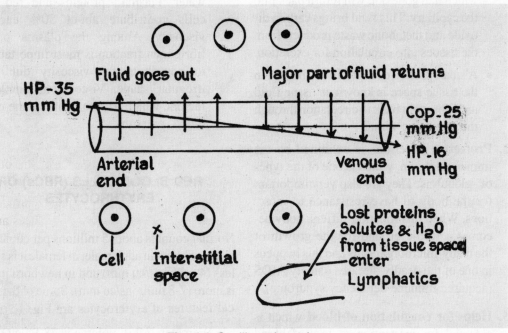

Fig. 1.2 Capillary dynamics

Capillary dynamics (Fig. 1.2):

Capillary has two different ends *a.* arterial end and *b.* venous end.

- The driving out force at the level of capillary will be the hydrostatic pressure exerted by the blood flowing through the capillary. This is about 35 mm Hg at the arterial end and 16 mm Hg at the venous end, because of decreased resistance by the wall of capillary at the venous end.

- Colliodal osmotic pressure will be the in-driving force at the capillary. This pressure opposes the hydrostatic pressure. Collidal osmotic pressure is around 25 mm Hg throughout the length of the capillary.

- Since the out-driving force is greater at the arterial end some amount of fluid goes out of the capillary into the tissue spaces. This fluid carries oxygen and nutrition to the tissues.

- At the venous end since the in-driving force is greater, a major part of the fluid which had gone out, will return back into the capillary. This fluid brings carbon dioxide and metabolic waste products from the tissues into circulation for excretion.

- A small portion of the fluid left behind in the tissue space is known as tissue fluid and is brought back to circulation through the lymphatic vessel.

2. **Protective function** is exhibited by the immunoglobulin, which is one of the types of globulins. They are also very important for the body to have resistance to infections. When this function suffers, body becomes a fertile ground for the growth of the many microorganisms and this happens in one of the deadly diseases namely AIDS (acquired immune deficiency syndrome).

3. **Helps for coagulation of blood** which is essential for prevention of loss of blood from any of the injured parts of the body. Most of the factors involved in coagulation of blood are plasma proteins in nature. Some of the important plasma proteins involved in coagulation are fibrinogen, prothrombin and antihemophilic globulin.

4. **Regulation of pH of blood:** The pH of blood has to be maintained within a critical range of 7.36 to 7.44 (7.4 ± 0.04) for the maintenance of normal body functions. The amino and carboxyl terminals of plasma proteins help to regulate pH of blood either by accepting or donating the H^+ and thereby prevent drastic variations in the pH of blood.

5. **Transport function:** Carbon dioxide gas, some of the metals like iron, copper and almost all the hormones are transported in the circulation to different parts of body by the plasma proteins.

6. **Maintenance of viscosity of blood:** Blood is 5-6 times more viscous than water. Plasma proteins and red blood cells contribute about 50% each for viscosity. Among the plasma proteins fibrinogen fraction is most important type to contribute for viscosity due to its irregular shape. Viscosity is one of the factors, which tries to maintain the normal blood pressure.

RED BLOOD CELLS (RBCs) OR ERYTHROCYTES

Normal count is about 5 millions per cubic millimetre of blood in adult male; in female it is slightly less (4 millions/cu mm) and in newborn infant it is more (7-8 millions/cu mm). Some of the physical features of erythrocytes are Fig. 1.2(a):

- Diameter: 7.2 µ, volume is 78-94 cu µ

- Shape is biconcave disc or dumbbell-shaped.
- Non-nucleated and contains hemoglobin.

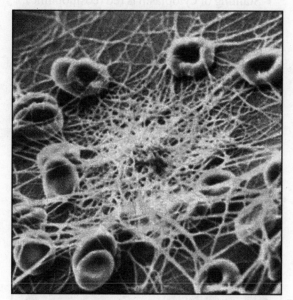

Fig 1.2(a) Electron microscopic view of RBCs

The functions of these cells are

- Transport of gases namely oxygen and carbon dioxide
- Regulation of pH of blood

All these functions are basically due to hemoglobin that is present in the cells.

The normal life span of the red blood cells is about 120 days.

They are produced in the red bone marrow and are destroyed in the reticuloendothelial tissue present in bone marrow, liver and spleen.

Erythrocyte sedimentation rate (ESR)

It is the rate at which erythrocytes settle down in unit time in a narrow pipette (Westergren's pipette). When red blood cells are allowed to settle down, a clear column of plasma will be at the top part of the pipette. The length of the plasma column will be taken as the ESR value.

The blood has to be treated with an ideal anticoagulant (3.8% sodium citrate solution) before blood is sucked into the pipette and allowed to sediment after fixing vertically to the stand and kept undisturbed for the next one hour.

Normal ESR value is about:

- 1-4 mm at the end of 1st hour in adult male
- 2-8 mm at the end of 1st hour in adult female
- < 1 mm at the end of 1st hour in children.

ESR is increased in many diseases and hence it does not have much significance as far as diagnosis of disease is concerned.

It has got more of prognostic value. On diagnosing the disease and after the start of the therapy, ESR is monitored periodically. If the therapy is working, then there will be gradual reduction in ESR value in course of time. One of the most common diseases in which ESR is increased is pulmonary tuberculosis.

ERYTHROPOIESIS

It is the process by which mature red blood cells are produced from the precursor stem cells. Normally it requires about 5-10 days. The three important sites from where erythropoiesis can take place are:

- Mesoderm of yolk sac in the first three months of fetal life (Mesoblastic stage).
- Liver and spleen during 3 – 6 months of fetal intrauterine life (Hepatic stage).
- From the red bone marrow in the rest of the period of the fetal life and in postnatal period (Myeloid stage).

In children red bone marrow is present in all the bones of the body. After the age of about 20 years it is restricted to all flat bones and proximal ends of long bones only.

Stages during erythropoiesis (Fig. 1.3)

Haemocytoblast (Stem Cell)

- Cell size – 20 – 24 μ
- Has nucleus and nucleoli
- No hemoglobin in the cytoplasm
- Staining of cytoplasm is blue (Basophilic)

Proerythroblast

- Cell size – 18 – 20 μ
- Has nucleus and nucleoli
- No hemoglobin in the cytoplasm
- Staining of cytoplasm is blue.

Early normoblast

- 16 – 18 μ
- Has nucleus and but not nucleoli
- No hemoglobin in the cytoplasm
- Staining of cytoplasm is blue.
- Mitosis occurs

Intermediate normoblast

- 12 – 14 μ
- Has nucleus
- Hemoglobin starts appearing.
- Hence the staining of cytoplasm is both blue and red (polychormatophillic).
- Mitosis occurs

Late normoblast

- 10 – 12 μ
- Has nucleus but the nucleus starts regressing and is lost ultimately
- The chromatin material appears from the regressing nucleus

- Hemoglobin content in the cytoplasm increases
- Staining of cytoplasm is red (eosinophilic).

Reticulocyte

- Size of the cell is slightly larger than red blood cell.
- The RNA still present in the cytoplasm can be shown by cresyl blue stain. The pattern of the distribution of RNA remnants varies.
- It takes about 24 – 48 hours for the reticulocyte to mature into an erythrocyte.
- Normal reticulocyte % in circulation is about 0 – 1 in adults. In children it is slightly more.

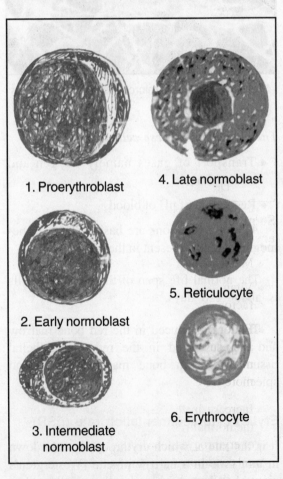

1. Proerythroblast   4. Late normoblast

2. Early normoblast   5. Reticulocyte

3. Intermediate normoblast   6. Erythrocyte

Fig. 1.3 Stages during erythropoiesis

The stimulus for erythropoiesis is Hypoxia. Hypoxia means a decrease in the oxygen supply to the tissues.

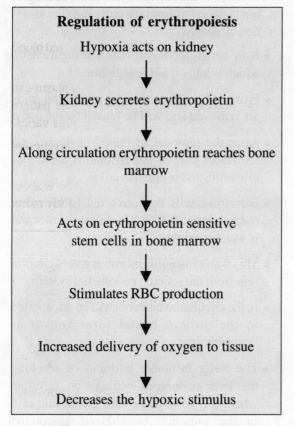

Regulation of erythropoiesis

Hypoxia acts on kidney

↓

Kidney secretes erythropoietin

↓

Along circulation erythropoietin reaches bone marrow

↓

Acts on erythropoietin sensitive stem cells in bone marrow

↓

Stimulates RBC production

↓

Increased delivery of oxygen to tissue

↓

Decreases the hypoxic stimulus

Some of the other factors influencing the erythropoiesis are:

- Metals like iron
- Vitamins like B_{12} and folic acid (maturation factors)
- Endocrine factors like thyroxin, androgens and estrogens. Androgen increases the formation of erythropoietin and hence slightly more RBC count in males than in females.

Increase in the red blood cell count above the normal range is known as polycythemia or erythrocytosis, occurs in certain pathological conditions like

- Chronic lung diseases

- Congenital heart diseases

And in physiological condition

- At high altitude (low barometric pressure area).

A decrease in cell count, called as oligocythemia, occurs in all types of anemia (pathological condition) and at below sea level (high barometric pressure area) in physiological condition.

HEMOGLOBIN

- This is the important pigment present in erythrocytes.
- It has got two parts namely the haem portion and globin part.
- Haem moiety is constituted by iron containing protoporphyrin rings and the proteins contribute globin part.
- Any hemoglobin molecule is made up of 4 polypeptide chains of proteins and the molecular weight is about 64500.

The difference in the polypeptide chains contributes for the different type of hemoglobin whereas the protoporphyrin rings remain the same in any type of hemoglobin.

There are two important types of hemoglobin.

- Hb A type has 2 α and 2 β chains and is present in adults.
- Hb F type has 2 α and 2 δ (delta) chains and is present in fetus.

The normal concentration of hemoglobin is about

- 14-18 g % in adult male
- 12-16 g % in adult female
- 18-22 g % in children

All the functions ascribed to RBCs are due this pigment. Each gram of hemoglobin has the ability to carry about 1.34 ml of oxygen. Oxygen is transported by the haem moiety and CO_2 is by the globin part.

Anemia is

- *Decrease in RBC count*
- *Or a decrease in hemoglobin concentration*
- *Or both*

Some of the common conditions in which anemia noticed are:

- Iron deficiency
- Depression of bone marrow
- Repeated blood loss (hemorrhage)
- Haemolysis.

Iron is one of the important raw materials required for hemoglobin synthesis and the daily requirement of iron is about 10 mg in adults.

Anemias can also be classified as (clinical classification)

- Hemolytic anemia *e.g.* malaria
- Deficiency anemias *e.g.* iron or vitamin B_{12} deficiency.
- Hemorrhagic anemia *e.g.* severe hemorrhage.

One of the popular methods of hemoglobin estimation is by Sahli's method, which is based on colorimetry.

When senile red blood cells are destroyed in the reticuloendothelial tissue, hemoglobin is metabolized and the pigment thus formed finally will be bilirubin.

Normally the bilirubin gets excreted from the body in the water-soluble form along with urine and faeces. Because of this, the bilirubin level in circulation is around 0.2 to 0.8 mg%.

Metabolism of hemoglobin

- After the senile red blood cells are destroyed in reticulo endothelial system, the hemoglobin is liberated from the cells and ring structure is altered.

- Now hemoglobin becomes a straight chain, which is known as choleglobin.

- From this choleglobin, iron and amino acids are removed and will be reused by the body.

- After the removal of these substances the remainder part of hemoglobin is known as biliverdin and is green in color.

- Bilivirdin will be converted to bilirubin (hemobilirubin), which is yellow in color and is water insoluble.

- This water insoluble bilirubin enters circulation from the reticulo endothelial system.

- In the circulation bilirubin will be transported in the protein bound form known as hemobilirubin.

- The water insoluble bilirubin on reaching the liver undergoes conjugation reaction, wherein it conjugates with glucuronic acid in the presence of enzyme glucuronyl transferase to form bilirubin glucuronide (cholebilirubin). Bilirubin glucuronide is water-soluble.

- It enters the small intestine along with bile.

- In the intestine the bacteria act upon the bilirubin and this results in the formation of bilinogens. Some amount of bilinogen get excreted along with the faeces (stercobilinogen). A lot of bilinogens reenter liver from intestine along the portal circulation, which ultimately get excreted from the body through kidneys in the form of urobilinogen.

- The bilinogens when exposed to the atmosphere will get converted to bilins.

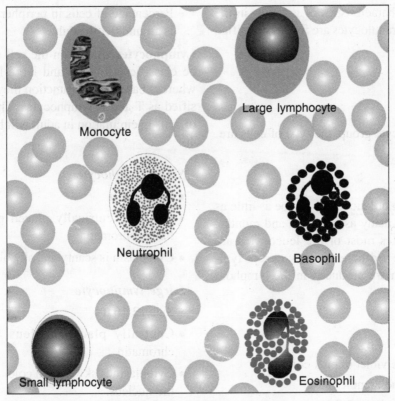

Fig 1.4 Morphology of WBCs

Jaundice

When the concentration of serum/plasma bilirubin exceeds 2 mg% it leads to condition namely jaundice. In jaundice there will be yellowish discoloration of

- Skin
- Mucous membrane
- Sclera of the eyes.

Increase in the bilirubin level may be due to

- Increased destruction of red blood cells by haemolysis (prehepatic/hemolytic jaundice)
- Improper functioning of liver (hepatic jaundice)
- Obstruction in biliary tract (post hepatic/obstructive jaundice).

WHITE BLOOD CELLS (WBCs) OR LEUCOCYTES

Leucocytes are the largest of all the formed elements in blood. Unlike red blood cells, which are non-nucleated cells, the white blood cells are nucleated. The number of leucocytes in circulation is around 4000 to 11000 cells per cu mm of blood in adults and in children it is about 18000 to 25000 cells/cu mm blood.

Depending on the presence or absence of granules in the cytoplasm, the leucocytes can be classified into

- Granulocytes
- Agranulocytes

Based on the staining property (Leishman

stain) and the characteristics of granules in the cytoplasm the granulocytes are further classified into

- Neutrophils
- Basophils
- Eosinophils

In the agranulocyte group, the type of cells are

- Lymphocyte
- Monocyte

The life span of leucocytes can be as little as few hours to as many as few days and months. Like erythrocytes most of the leucocytes are produced in the red bone marrow except lymphocytes, which are produced in the lymphoid tissue.

Neutrophil

- Cell size 10-14 μ
- Granules are violet or pink colored
- Plenty of fine granules
- Nucleus may have 2-7 lobes
- Percentage of cells in peripheral circulation is around 40-70 in adult.

Eosinophil

- Cell size 10-14 μ
- Granules appear red colored
- Few, coarse and compactly packed granules
- Nucleus is usually bi lobed
- Percentage of cells in peripheral circulation is around 1-6 in adult.

Basophil

- Cell size 10-14 μ
- Granules are dark blue colored
- Very few coarse granules
- Nucleus is usually bilobed and since the staining of the nucleus and granules is same, most of the times the nucleus gets masked.

- Percentage of cells in peripheral circulation is around 0-1 in adult.

Lymphocytes: Based on the cell size they can be classified as small and large lymphocytes, whereas based on the function they can be classified as T and B lymphocytes. The percentage of cells in circulation in adult will be around 25-40.

Small lymphocyte

- Size 8-10 μ
- Large eccentrically placed nucleus with lumpy chromatin
- Cytoplasm is scanty and sky blue in color.

Large lymphocyte

- Size 12-16 μ
- Centrally placed nucleus with lumpy chromatin
- Cytoplasm is sky blue in color and encircles the nucleus.

Monocyte

- Size 16-21 μ
- Kidney- or horseshoe-shaped nucleus with reticular chromatin
- Cytoplasm appears muddy grey or frosted glass-like
- Percentage of cells in circulation will be around 2-8.

Functions

Neutrophils and monocytes provide non-specific or innate immunity and is directed against bacteria only. They provide immunity by a mechanism known as phagocytosis.

The steps in phagocytosis are

- Margination
- Diapedesis

- +ve chemotaxis
- Phagocytosis proper
- Digestion

Margination

White blood cells are in the central stream of blood flow in the vascular region, and come to the margin of the vessel wall when blood flows through the area of infection. This is because as the blood vessel will have got dilated at the site of infection, vasodilation leads to reduction in the velocity of blood flow.

Diapedesis

The cells put forth pseudopodia like structures and make their way from the intravascular compartment to interstitial spaces across the vascular wall. The process of movement of cells from intravascular to extra vascular regions is known as emigration.

+ve Chemotaxis

The chemical substances (chemoattractants) liberated by the invaded bacteria will attract the leucocytes towards themselves, which is termed as positive chemotaxis. If the toxins liberated by

bacteria are very strong (virulent), the leucocytes get repelled away from the bacteria. This is known as –ve chemotaxis.

Phagocytosis proper

The pseudopodia like process put out by the leucocytes will completely encircle the bacteria and the bacteria are engulfed by the leucocytes.

Digestion

The proteolytic and lipolytic enzymes and lysozymes released by the leucocytes will digest the bacteria.

Increase in the neutrophil % is known as neutrophilia and occurs in any acute pyogenic (pus forming) infections like appendicitis, tonsillitis. Neutrophil % decrease is known as neutropenia which is seen in typhoid, paratyphoid, malaria.

Monocyte % is increased (monocytosis) in tuberculosis, syphilis.

Specific immunity (Schematic Chart 1.1)

This is being provided by the lymphocytes. As stated earlier the lymphocytes can be classified as T and B types based on the function.

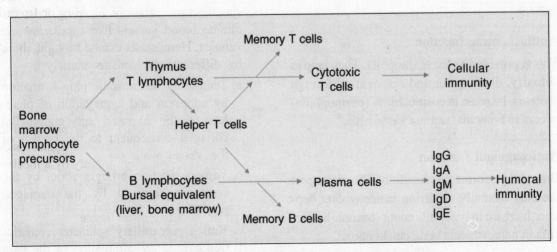

Schematic chart 1.1 - indicating the specific immunity

The T lymphocytes

- Provide cellular immunity
- Cellular immunity is normally against bacteria, viruses, fungi and parasites and also against the tissues/organs that are transplanted.
- 80% of lymphocytes in peripheral circulation belong to this group.

The B type lymphocyte

- Provide humoral immunity
- Humoral immunity is only against bacteria and the free antibodies in circulation are gamma globulins in nature.
- 20% lymphocytes belong to this type

The precursor cells of lymphocytes get migrated from bone marrow to either thymus or to any of the other region lymph nodes. If the precursor cell gets processed in thymus, then it develops into T lymphocyte and if gets processed in any other region lymph nodes lead to the production of B-lymphocytes.

Increase in lymphocyte percentage is termed lymphocytosis occurs in chronic conditions like syphilis.

Antihistaminic function

This is provided by the eosinophils. They help to detoxify, disintegrate and removal of foreign proteins. Increase in eosinophil % (eosinophilia) occurs in bronchial asthma, dermatitis.

Anticoagulant function

Basophil performs this function. They transport the only naturally occurring anticoagulant heparin. Increase in basophils count (basophilia) occurs in polycythemia vera, chickenpox.

When leucocyte count is above the normal range it is known as Leucocytosis seen in acute pyogenic infections like tonsillitis, appendicitis and a decrease in the cell count is known as Leucopenia seen in typhoid, paratyphoid.

PLATELETS (THROMBOCYTES)

- Size is about 2-4 μ
- Non-nucleated circular or oval shaped bodies
- On treating with ammonium oxalate they appear as shining bodies
- Life span is about 7 days and these cells are produced from megakaryocytes present in the red bone marrow.
- They get destroyed in spleen. Hence in splenomegaly the cell count decreases (thrombocytopenia). Increase in thrombocyte count (Thrombocytosis) occurs in accidents, after delivery, following surgical operations, fractures.
- The normal count is around 150000 to 450000 per cu mm of blood.

Functions of platelets

1. **Haemostasis:** One of the important functions being haemostasis. It means the spontaneous arrest of bleeding from the minute blood vessels like capillaries and venules. Hemostasis can be brought about by different mechanisms namely:

   a. Temporary haemostatic plug formation by adhesion and aggregation of platelets to the exposed sub endothelial collagen consequent to the breach of the vessel wall.

   b. Vasoconstriction brought about by the serotonin released by the damaged platelets.

   c. Reflex precapillary sphincter constriction caused by stimulation of the pain receptors at the site of injury.

d. Accumulation of fluid in the tissue spaces at the site of injury may increase the pressure around the vessel wall and exert a compressor force on the wall of blood vessel.

2. **Blood coagulation:** The phospholipid substance released by damaged platelets will help in the formation of prothrombin activator in the intrinsic system of blood coagulation.

3. **Clot retraction:** The decrease in the size of clot as the time elapses and the change in the texture of clot is due to clot retraction. Clot retraction is aided by a protein present in platelets namely thrombasthenin.

4. **Phagocytosis:** The immune complexes, carbon particles are phagocytosed.

Purpura

- Hemorrhagic spots seen below the skin, mucus membrane.
- This occurs especially in thrombocytopenia
- In purpura the bleeding time is increased, but clotting time remains normal.
- The normal bleeding time is about 1-4 min.
- The definition of bleeding time is interval from the onset of bleeding till the spontaneous arrest of bleeding from the capillaries.
- In hemophilia bleeding time will be normal.

COAGULATION OR CLOTTING OF BLOOD

The conversion of fluid blood into semisolid jelly like mass is known as coagulation or clotting of blood. The process of clotting involves a number of substances, which are called factors.

There are 3 basic steps in the coagulation of blood:

- Formation of prothrombin activator
- Conversion of prothrombin to thrombin
- Conversion of fibrinogen to fibrin and clot formation

Two mechanisms which can bring about the formation of prothrombin activator are

- Intrinsic mechanism/system
- Extrinsic mechanism/system

In intrinsic mechanism all the factors required for this reactions are present in blood itself and in extrinsic mechanism the factors present in blood and some coming from damaged tissue are contributing. But for the first step (prothrombin activator formation), all the other steps (conversion of prothrombin to thrombin and fibrinogen to fibrin) are common for both intrinsic and extrinsic mechanisms of blood clotting.

Factor No.	Name
I	Fibrinogen
II	Prothrombin
III	Tissue thromboplastin (TF)
IV	Ca^{++}
V	Proaccelerin
VI	ABSENT
VII	Proconvertin
VIII	Antihemophilic factor
IX	Christmas factor
X	Stuart Prower factor
XI	Plasma thromboplastin antecedent
XII	Hageman's factor
XIII	Fibrin stabilizing factor

In addition to the above some of the other factors that have role in coagulation of blood are Kallekrien, High molecular weight kininogen, Von Willebrandt factor.

Schematic chart of blood coagulation details are as per chart 1.2. In the chart, both the intrinsic and extrinsic mechanisms steps have been indicated.

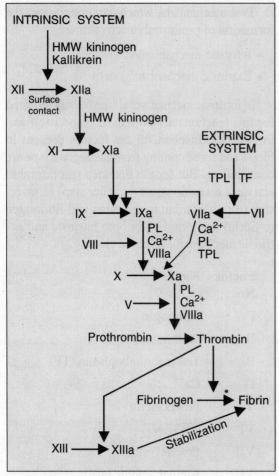

Schematic chart 1.2 – indicating steps in coagulation of blood

The steps of coagulation have three special features viz. (a) enzyme substrate reaction, (b) bioamplifier system, and (c) cascade reaction.

In enzyme substrate reaction the active form of the factor acts as an enzyme and acts on the next inactive factor (substrate) to activate it. (For e.g. factor XIIa acts as enzyme to activate factor XI (substrate) to XIa

In bioamplifier system small quantity of earlier factor have the ability to activate large quantity of the next factor.

Cascade reaction is one in which the rate of reaction goes on increasing along the steps.

The definition of clotting time is time interval from the onset of bleeding till the formation of clot (fibrin threads).

- It is usually estimated by capillary method in the laboratory
- Normal clotting time is about 4-8 min.
- It is increased in conditions like hemophilia, Christmas disease, afibrinogenemia and prothrombanemia.

Anticoagulants are substances, which have the ability to prevent the clotting of blood.

Anticoagulants can be classified into

- In Vitro
- In Vivo

In vivo anticoagulants are (which are used inside the body)

- Heparin
- Dicumorol

The in vitro anticoagulants are (which are used outside the body)

- Sodium citrate 3.8% solution.
- Double oxalate (oxalate of K^+ and ammonium)
- Heparin
- EDTA (ethylene diamine tetra acetic acid)

Anticoagulants are used to

- Store blood in blood bank
- Maintain fluid state of blood while doing certain tests in the laboratory

• As therapeutic agent to prevent intravascular clotting (thrombosis).

Mechanism of action

Heparin exhibits anticoagulant effect by exerting :

• Antithrombin actions

• Antithromboplastin effect

• And also by preventing the aggregation of platelets.

Dicumarol acts as a competitive inhibitor for vitamin K that is essential for the synthesis of the clotting factors No. II, VII, IX and X by the liver.

The inorganic salts (sodium citrate, double oxalate, EDTA) act as anticoagulant either by precipitating or chelating the ionic calcium that is essential for clotting of blood.

Clot retraction

• Freshly formed clot is soft and big.

• As the time progresses not only the size of clot decreases but also the texture of the clot is altered.

• The clot becomes harder

• The normal clot retraction ratio is about 40-60% to the original size after the first hour.

• The fluid part that is squeezed out during clot retraction is called as serum

• Serum is identical to plasma in all aspects except for the absence of factor No. I, II, V, VIII and XIII.

Fibrinolysis

The process of breakdown of clot is known as fibrinolysis and the system involved is known as fibrinolytic system. Plasminogen is present in the circulating plasma and at the time of fibrinolysis this is converted to active form plasmin (either by intrinsic/extrinsic mechanism). This plasmin acts on the clot and brings about the lysis of the clot and ultimately the fibrin degradation products are formed. This helps to remove millions of minute clots, which may be getting formed during the circulation of blood. If these clots are not removed they may clog the blood vessel and lead to ischemia of the tissues.

Hemophilia (classical hemophilia or hemophilia A)

• It is a sex-linked disease.

• Due to deficiency of factor No. VIII.

• The gene is present on X chromosome

• Normally the males suffer and females act as the carriers (as male has only one X chromosome with the recessive gene whereas the female has two X chromosomes one with normal gene and one carrying the recessive gene).

• These patients will have a prolonged clotting time, but normal bleeding time.

• At times they may have severe bleeding even from a minute injury.

• The common symptom is painful swollen joints.

Christmas disease: Which is also known as hemophilia B and is due to the absence of factor no. IX. It is not that severe like the classical hemophilia.

BLOOD GROUPS

On the red blood cells there can be the presence of certain agglutinogens or antigens. The presence or absence of the group specific agglutinogen on these cells forms the basis of blood grouping. The biochemical nature of the agglutinogen in general is glycoprotein or mucopolysaccharide.

There are different systems of blood grouping and the agglutinogen considered in each system is specific. Some of the major systems of blood grouping are

- ABO system and agglutinogens considered will be A & B
- Rh system and agglutinogen considered will be D
- MN system and agglutinogens considered will be M & N

In plasma there may be presence of certain substances namely agglutinins or antibodies. Corresponding agglutinins act against specific agglutinogens. When an agglutinogen reacts with specific agglutinin it leads to a reaction called agglutination or clumping.

Based on the presence or absence of this group specific agglutinogen on the red blood cell the blood grouping can be done as follows:

ABO SYSTEM		
Agglutinogen on RBC	Agglutinin in plasma	Blood group
A present	Anti B (β)	A
B present	Anti A (α)	B
A & B present	both absent	AB
A & B absent	both present (α and β)	O

Rh SYSTEM		
Agglutinogen on RBC	Agglutinin in plasma	Blood group
D present	Nil	Rh^+
D absent	Nil	Rh^-

The antibodies belonging to ABO system are known as naturally occurring antibodies whereas the Rh antibodies are produced only when Rh negative person is transfused with Rh positive blood.

Based on the observation of the agglutinogen and agglutinin present in a person's blood, Karl Landsteiner stated the following law.

The 1st part of the law states that when a particular agglutinogen is present on the red blood cells the corresponding agglutinin must be absent in the plasma.

The 2nd part of the law is when a particular agglutinogen is absent on the red blood cells the corresponding agglutinin will be present in the plasma.

- ABO system obeys both the parts of the law
- Rh system and all other systems of blood grouping obey the first part of law only.

Agglutinogens of different systems may coexist. Hence we can come across all permutations and combinations in the blood group of individuals which can be

A^+,	A^-,
B^+,	B^-,
AB^+	AB^-
O^+	O^-

Determination of blood group

Procedure

- A drop of known antiserum (agglutinin) is taken on the slide.
- To this add a drop of cell suspension (drop of blood and 1 ml of 0.9 % sodium chloride solution).
- Mix well.
- The slide should be placed on a wet filter paper and covered with petri dish.
- Wait for a minimum of 10 minutes
- At the end of 10 minutes the slide is observed for agglutination reaction with the naked eye and then under the microscope.

OBSERVATION	CONCLUSION
In ABO system agglutination with	*Blood group will be*
Anti-A serum only	A
Anti-B serum only	B
Both in anti-A and anti-B sera	AB
None of the sera	O

In the same way the Rh system will also be determined using anti D antibodies.

Importance of blood grouping

- Done mainly for blood transfusion purposes.

- Is also important in certain medico legal aspects as well. Blood group specific agglutinogen may also appear in certain secretions like saliva. People in whom the agglutinogen is present in bodily secretions are called secretors.

- In anthropological studies as well (geographical distribution of races)

- In disputed paternity also to ascertain who is not the father of the child.

Cross matching

Before any transfusion it is very important to ascertain whether the donor and recipient blood match.

There are two types of cross matching

- Major cross matching
- Minor cross matching

In major cross matching the donor's cell suspension is matched with recipient's plasma. In minor cross matching it is donor's plasma with recipient's cell suspension is matched.

If there is agglutination, the groups are considered to be not matching or incompatible.

Table of compatibility				
Recipient *Donor*	*A*	*B*	*AB*	*O*
A	–	+	–	+
B	+	–	–	+
AB	+	+	–	+
O	–	–	–	–

– sign denotes compatibility (matching)
+ sign incompatibility (not matching).

AB positive persons are universal recipients and O negative individuals are universal donors.

Different types of transfusion and condition in which it is done:

- Whole blood in hemorrhage
- Erythrocytes alone in severe anemia
- Only plasma in burns
- Only leucocytes in severe leucopoenia
- Only platelets in severe thrombocytopenia.
- Exchange transfusion in erythroblastosis fetalis.

Hazards of blood transfusion

a. *Compatible blood transfusion*

- Transmission of diseases like AIDS, syphilis, malaria.
- Overloading of heart.
- Ionic imbalances if stored blood is not brought to room temperature before transfusion.
- Patient may develop fever, shivering, rigors due to bacterial toxins.

b. *Incompatible blood transfusion*

- The extent of reaction depends on the severity of the situation.

- **Minor** - there can be inapparent hemolysis due to which after one or two days of transfusion the serum bilirubin level may go up to as much as 1.2 mg %
- **Moderate** - in which patient develops jaundice due to increase in the bilirubin level beyond 2 mg%.
- **Severe** - the agglutinated mass of cells may block circulation in the capillaries, which lead to pain in the chest and back. If the agglutinated mass blocks the renal circulation the patient develops kidney failure. The loss of kidney function leads to increase in blood urea, creatinine levels and may damage the brain.

Erythroblastosis foetalis

- This is a condition of the newborn infant.
- It develops due to the incompatibility between the Rh blood group of the mother and the fetus.
- The blood group of mother will be Rh negative and that of fetus will be Rh positive.
- Normally there is no problem with the first pregnancy as there will be no naturally occurring anti D antibodies.
- At the time of delivery some of the Rh positive cells of the fetus enter maternal circulation and stimulate the immune system of mother to produce anti D antibodies (sensitize the immune system).
- In subsequent pregnancies if the fetus happens to be Rh positive, chances are there that the antibodies are produced in the mother's body in large amounts.
- Since these antibodies can cross the placental barrier as they belong to Ig G group (unlike the ABO group antibodies which belong to Ig M group and can't cross placenta), they enter the fetal circulation and bring about the hemolysis of the fetal red blood cells.

This is a very serious situation. In such a situation the newborn infant will be given exchange transfusion and the type of blood preferred will be O negative.

Inheritance of blood group (Schematic Chart 1.3)

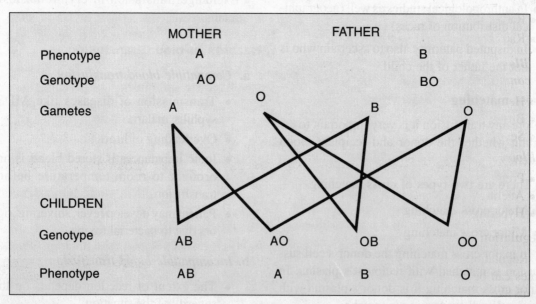

Schematic chart 1.3 – inheritance of blood group from parents who have heterozygous genotype

- The group specific genes are present on the autosomes and are dominant genes.
- Even if the gene is present on one of the pairs of the chromosome the particular group is inherited.
- One of the genes will be inherited from the mother and the other from the father.
- For example in person whose blood group is A, the genotype of the individual may be homozygous (AA) or heterozygous (AO) state. Like that it can be with B group also. But for O group person the genotype will always be OO and AB group person it will be AB only.

BLOOD VOLUME AND LYMPH

Blood volume

As stated at the beginning the normal blood volume in a normal adult male is about 5 litres or 70-ml/kg-body weight. Blood volume can be determined based on the principle of dilution. Some of the substances used are

- Evans blue
- Radioactive iodine
- Radioactive chromium.

Blood volume decreases (hypovolemia) in conditions like

- Hemorrhage
- Burns
- Severe vomiting, diarrhea

Blood volume is increased in

- Pregnancy
- Anemia
- Hyperthyroidism.

Regulation of blood volume

Regulation of blood volume in hypovolemic states can be brought about by various mechanisms like

- Fluid shift (alterations in the forces acting at

the level of capillary which is responsible for movement of fluid from the tissue spaces into the intravascular compartment).

- Thirst
- Concentration of urine
- Increased secretion of hormones like ADH/vasopressin, aldosterone.

Functions of spleen

- Erythropoiesis in fetal life
- Destruction of senile red blood cells and platelets
- Production of lymphocytes and antibodies
- Storage of blood in lower animals

Functions of lymph nodes

- Production of lymphocytes
- Production of antibodies
- Act as a filter for the bacteria so that they are confined to lymph nodes only.

Lymph

This is nothing but the tissue fluid that has entered the lymphatic vessel. The formation of lymph can be explained based on the capillary dynamics (refer maintenance of colloidal osmotic pressure under plasma proteins functions).

Functions of lymph:

- Transport of fluid and lost proteins from tissue spaces back into circulation.
- Transport of lymphocytes and antibodies into circulation from the lymph nodes.
- Transport of absorbed lipids from the intestine.
- Transport of proteins from liver into circulation.

Any obstruction in the lymphatic drainage will lead to increased fluid accumulation in the tissue spaces and gives rise to edema. Elephantiasis or filariasis is one of the commonest diseases in which drainage of lymph is blocked.

Renal Physiology

- Introduction
- Nephron and filtration
- Reabsorption and secretion
- Concentration of urine
- Juxta glomerular apparatus.
- Micturition
- Cystometrogram
- Composition of urine
- Skin and thermoregulation

INTRODUCTION

Renal physiology deals with the study of structure and functions of the excretory system. The parts included in this system are

a. Pair of kidneys
b. Pair of ureters

c. Urinary bladder and
d. Urethra

The primary function of the renal system is to maintain the constancy of the internal environment (Homeostasis).

Homeostasis includes the regulation of

- Osmolarity of plasma
- Volume of plasma
- Electrolytes concentration
- Excretion of metabolic wastes
- Secretion of certain hormones like
  a. erythropoietin
  b. active form of vitamin D.
- Acid base balance of the body.

Normal weight of each of the kidney is about 150 g and both the kidneys together receive an average of 1200 ml of blood per minute.

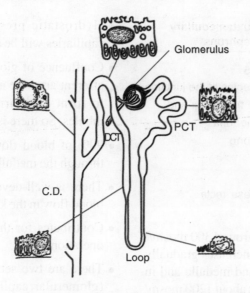

Fig 2 .1 Structure of nephron

STRUCTURE AND FUNCTIONAL ASPECTS OF NEPHRON

Nephron is the structural and functional unit of kidney. In each kidney there are about 1 million nephrons.

Each nephron is made up of two different parts (Fig. 2.1)
- *Renal corpuscle*
- *Renal tubules*

The glomerular capillaries and Bowman's capsule constitute the renal corpuscle.

The parts of renal tubules are
- Proximal convoluted tubule (PCT)
- Loop of Henle (LH)
- Distal convoluted tubule (DCT)
- Collecting duct

There are two different types of nephrons (Fig. 2.2). One of the types is known as cortical and the other as juxtamedullary nephron.

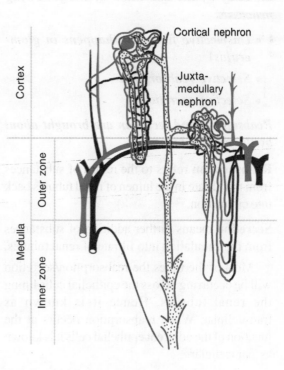

Fig 2.2 Types of nephron

Cortical nephrons	Juxtamedullary nephrons
% of nephrons 85	15
Most of the parts of nephron are in cortex only	Begins at the junction of the cortex and medulla
Length of LH short	Long
Accompanied by peritubular capillary network	Vasa recta

The interstitial osmolarity is around 300 mosm/l of water in the cortex and it increases gradually from the junction of cortex and medulla and in the deepest part of medulla it is about 1200 mosm/l of water.

The kidney brings about the homeostasis of the body by the operation of the following processes.

- *Unselective filtration (happens in glomerulus)*
- *Selective reabsorption*
- *Selective secretion*

Reabsoption and secretion are brought about by the renal tubules.

Reabsorption refers to the return of substances from the filtrate in the lumen of renal tubules back into circulation.

Secretion means further addition of substances from the circulation into filtrate of renal tubules.

Most of the times the reabsorption/secretion will be occurring across the epithelial cells lining the renal tubules. Hence it is known as transcellular. When reabsorption occurs at the junction of the adjacent epithelial cells it is known as paracellular.

Renal circulation: Some of the special features

- Normal blood flow is about 1200 ml/min

- Hydrostatic pressure in the glomerular capillaries will be as high as 45 mm Hg.
- Confluence of glomerular capillaries forms efferent arteriole and this arteriole branches to form capillaries accompanying renal tubules. So there is portal circulation.
- 90% of blood flows through cortex, 7-9% through the medulla.
- There is well-developed auto regulation of blood flow in the kidney.
- Contributes for the counter current system operation.
- There are two sets of capaillaries. One set (glomerular capillaries) for filtration and another set (capillaries accompanying renal tubules) for reabsorption/secretion.
- Cell lining of arteriole contributes for the formation of juxtaglomerular apparatus.

Renal fraction is the ratio of cardiac output that flows into the kidneys. Normally it is about 25 %. The renal blood flow can be measured by *applying Fick's principle*. The substance normally used to measure renal blood flow is PAH (para amino hippuric acid). The renal plasma flow will be about 700 ml and the renal blood flow will be 1200 ml/min.

GLOMERULAR FILTRATION

Glomerular Filtration Rate (GFR)

It is the rate at which the filtration occurs in all the two million nephrons per minute. Normal value is about 125 ml/min ± 10 ml or 180 L/day. In female it is about 10% less than in males.

The type of filtration occurs in the kidney is known as *ultrafiltration as all substances present in plasma get filtered except plasma proteins.*

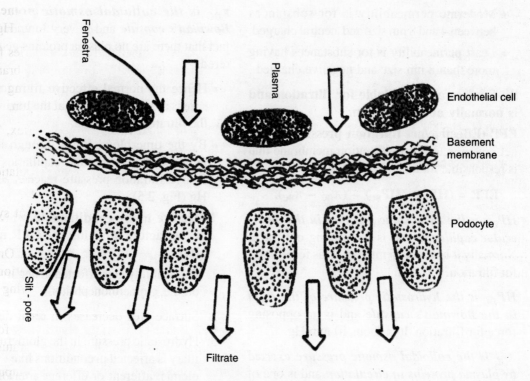

Fig 2.3 Structure of filtration membrane

Filtration fraction is the ratio between the glomerular filtration rate and renal plasma flow.

Normally it is 0.16-0.2.

Factors affecting/responsible for GFR

GFR = K, S, EFP

- K – Permeability constant of filtration membrane.
- S – Surface area available for filtration.
- EFP – Effective (net) filtration pressure.

K is the permeability constant. Permeability of the substance across the filtration membrane is *not only influenced by the molecular size of the substance but also on the charge the substance carries* (Figs. 2.3 and 2.4).

- Maximum permeability is for substances of less than 4 nm size and positively charged.

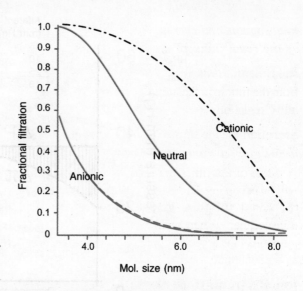

Fig 2.4 Factors influencing permeability across the membrane

- Moderate permeability is for substances between 4 and 8 nm size and neutral charged.
- Least permeability is for substances having more than 8 nm size and negative charged.

S—Surface area available for filtration and is normally about 0.8 sq m.

EFP (Effective/net filtration pressure) is the net pressure across the filtration membrane that is responsible for the ultrafiltration.

$$EFP = (HP_{GC} - HP_{BC}) - (\pi_{GC} - \pi_{BC}).$$

HP_{GC} *is the hydrostatic pressure in the glomerular capillaries* and is the driving out force. Normally it is about 45 mm Hg. This force helps for filtration.

HP_{BC} *is the hydrostatic pressure of the fluid in the Bowman's capsule* and is an opposing force for filtration. It is about 10 mm Hg.

π_{GC} *is the colloidal osmotic pressure exerted by plasma proteins in circulation* and is one of the forces that opposes filtration. Normally it is about 25 mm Hg.

π_{BC} *is the colloidal osmotic pressure in Bowman's capsule* and is very low, due to the fact that there are no plasma proteins getting filtered.

- Hence the normal effective filtration pressure is around 10 mm Hg at the beginning of the filtration membrane.
- By the time blood flows through half the length of the glomerular capillaries the effective filtration pressure reaches zero mm Hg (Fig. 2.5).

There are many conditions in which each of the factors affecting the GFR may get altered.

1. Permeability gets affected in nephrotic syndrome, glomerulonephritis.

2. Surface area decreases in renal diseases.

3. Hydrostatic pressure in the glomerular capillary is affected in conditions like hypovolemia, afferent or efferent arteriolar constriction.

4. Colloidal osmotic pressure in the circulation

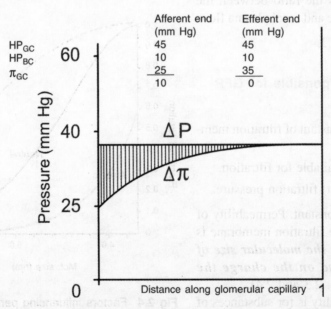

	Afferent end (mm Hg)	Efferent end (mm Hg)
HP_{GC}	45	45
HP_{BC}	10	10
π_{GC}	25	35
	10	0

Fig 2.5 Effective filtration pressure across the membrane and equilibration point

gets affected in liver diseases, kidney diseases, haemodilution and haemo-concentration.

5. Hydrostatic pressure in Bowman's capsule is increased in edema of kidney (hydronephrosis) or because of obstruction in the urinary tract (renal stones).

Apart from the aforesaid factors, which can alter the GFR, one of the other important factors is the renal blood flow. But the blood flow to the kidney has got a well-developed auto regulation. Because of this the blood flow to the kidney is normally maintained constant between a pressure ranges of 60 and 160 mm Hg. The maintenance of blood flow constant can be explained based on

- Myogenic
- Renin angiotensin
- Tissue metabolite and
- Interstitial fluid pressure theories.

Clearance concept

- It is the volume of plasma losing (getting cleared off) a particular substance in one minute.

- The substance from the plasma can enter the renal tubules by a process of filtration.

- Substance that has reached the tubules may either get back to circulation by a process of reabsorption or can get added on further into the renal tubules by a process of secretion.

- For any substance to get lost from the plasma the prerequisite is, it should get filtered. It is for this reason the plasma proteins do not have clearance value as plasma proteins don't get filtered.

$$\text{Clearance value} = \frac{U \times V}{P}$$

U= concentration of substance in urine (mg/ml).

P= concentration of substance in plasma (mg/ml)

V= volume of urine formed per minute (ml/min)

Normal clearance value for some of the important substances is **(ml/min)**

Inulin	125
Urea	70
Glucose	0
Creatinine	140
PAH	630

When clearance value of any substance is

- *Less than 125 ml/min means the substance is getting reabsorbed partially or completely*

- *125 ml/min means the substance is neither reabsorbed nor secreted*

- *More than 125 ml/min means the substance is getting secreted partially or completely.*

Determination of GFR

- *Determination of glomerular filtration rate provides some information regarding the functional status of the kidneys.*

- *Inulin can be used to determine GFR as it obeys the following criteria:*

a. Is freely filtred

b. Neither reabsorbed nor secreted

c. Doesn't get metabolized in the body

d. Doesn't alter the blood flow to the kidney

e. Non-toxic

f. Can be accurately estimated from a sample of urine

- *In clinical practice normally the creatinine clearance value is considered, as this substance is endogenously produced unlike inulin, which has to be injected into the body in a controlled way while determining GFR.*

Renal Threshold

It is the concentration of substance in plasma (mg%) at or above which it starts getting excreted in urine.

Tubular / transport maximum

It is the maximum ability of renal tubules either to reabsorb or secrete any substance in one minute (mg/min).

Reabsorption of substances in renal tubules can be brought about by any of the following mechanisms:

- Passive reabsorption *is where the reabsorption is along the electrical / concentration gradient or both. Energy is not required here.*

- Active reabsorption *is where the reabsorption occurs against the electrical / concen-*

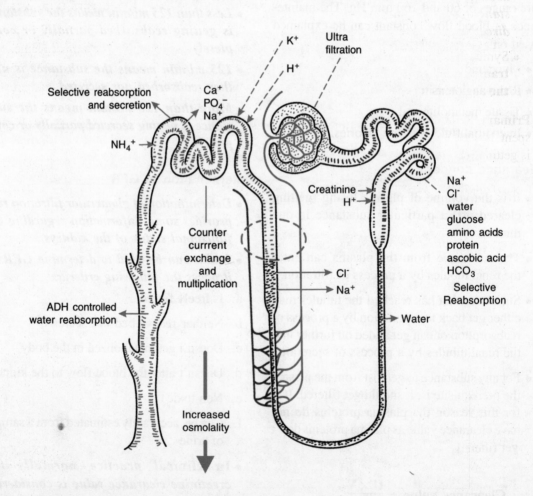

Fig 2.6 Reabsorption of various substances in different parts of renal tubules

tration gradient or both. This type of re-absorption requires the expenditure of energy.

- Simple diffusion *wherein there is movement of substances across the cell through the special pores / channels.*
- Carrier mediated *wherein the substance bind to special protein molecules on the cell membrane during their movement into the cell.*

Carrier mediated may be

- Antiport / counter transport – *which brings about the transport of two different substances by the same carrier in opposing directions.*
- Symport / Co-transport – **which helps in transport of two different substances by the same carrier in the same direction.**

Primary active transport means the energy spent is directly related to the substance that is getting reabsorbed. E.g Sodium reabsorption.

Secondary active transport means the energy spent for the reabsorption of some substance help in reabsorption of certain other substance. E.g. Glucose reabsorption (secondary active transport) is due to the primary active reabsorption of sodium.

While reabsorption movement of substances can be

- Across the cell (transcellular)
  Or
- At the junction of the adjacent cells (paracellular).

Sodium reabsorption occurs (Fig. 2.7)

- In almost all the parts of tubules except in the descending limb of loop of Henle.
- Basically by primary active transport.
- By symport or antiport mechanisms to a greater extent.
- In distal convoluted tubule also and is influenced by the hormones aldosterone, atrial natriuretic peptide.

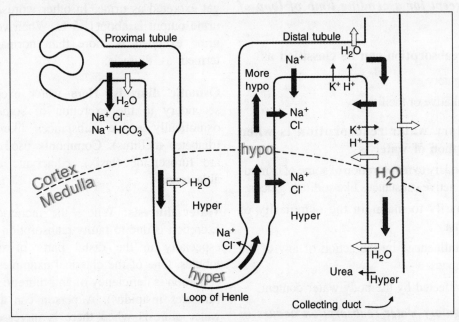

Fig 2.7 Sodium reabsorption in different parts and associated other substances movement

Glucose reabsorption

- Occurs only in proximal convoluted tubule.
- Is brought about by symport mechanism.
- The substance cotransported will be sodium.
- The reabsorption of glucose is by a secondary active transport as the energy spent for sodium reabsorption helps in binding of sodium to the carrier protein, which in turn facilitates the binding of glucose to the carrier.
- Normally glucose is not excreted in the urine and hence the glucose clearance value is 0 ml/min.
- **When glucose gets excreted in the urine the condition is known as glycosuria.** Glucose starts getting excreted when blood glucose level exceeds the renal threshold of 180 mg%.
- One of the common conditions in which glycosuria occurs is in diabetes mellitus.
- The tubular maximum for glucose is 375 mg/min.

Water reabsorption occurs in all parts of tubules except for ascending limb of loop of Henle.

Water reabsorption can be classified as

- Obligatory
- Facultative or facilitatory

Obligatory water reabsorption is when reabsorption of water is

- Secondary to reabsorption of some of osmotically active substances like sodium, glucose.
- Primarily to maintain the osmolarity of plasma.
- Not influenced by the action of any of the hormones.
- Not affected by the body water content.

Obligatory water reabsorption occurs in proximal convoluted tubule only.

Facultative / Facilitatory water reabsorption occurs

- In the distal convoluted tubules and collecting ducts.
- Here water reabsorption is independent of reabsorption of the other substances.
- The increase in the reabsorption will be due to the insertion of the water channels into the epithelial cells by the action of anti-diuretic hormone .
- In the absence of this hormone there will be abnormal increase in the urine output, which can be as high as 22 L/day as against a normal value of 1-1.5 L/day.
- This type of diuresis is known as water diuresis.
- The extent of water reabsorbed is less when the body water content is more.

Diuresis means an increased volume of urine output. Normally out of 125 ml of plasma gets filtered per minute, only 1 ml or even less will get excreted as urine. In other words, per day urine output is about 1.5 L. When volume of urine excreted is more than normal this is termed as diuresis.

Osmotic diuresis: Here water excretion is secondary to the excretion of some of the osmotically active substances like glucose (diabetes mellitus). Commonly used diuretics are furosemide (lasix), ethacrynic acid and aldactone.

Water diuresis: Where the increased water excretion is due to faulty reabsorption of water especially in the distal parts of the renal tubules. One of the classical examples for this condition is deficiency of anti diuretic hormone (diabetes insipidus). A person can also have water diuresis when there is increased water intake.

Bicarbonate reabsorption

Almost all the filtered bicarbonate is

- Reabsorbed in the proximal convoluted tubule.
- Diffused into the cells from the tubular lumen as carbon dioxide.
- H^+ is secreted into the lumen by antiport mechanism.
- In the lumen bicarbonate reacts with H^+ secreted by the cells to form carbonic acid, which in turn dissociates to carbon dioxide and water. For this reaction to occur carbonic anhydrase enzyme is necessary and is present at the brush border of the epithelial cells.
- On entering the cells carbon dioxide again reacts with water in presence of carbonic anhydrase of the cell to form carbonic acid and this dissociates to form H^+ and bicarbonate.
- The bicarbonate diffuses into circulation ultimately.

Potassium

- The filtered potassium is reabsorbed in the proximal convoluted tubule.
- Whatever potassium that appears in the urine comes from the distal convoluted tubules, as the distal convoluted tubules secrete potassium ion in exchange for sodium ion that is reabsorbed.

Calcium reabsorption in the distal convoluted tubules is under the influence of action of hormones namely parathormone and calcitonin.

Urea

- Reabsorption occurs mostly in the proximal tubules.
- However the amount of urea reabsorbed is limited when compared to other substances.

- Hence the urea clearance value is about 70 ml/min.
- There is some amount of recycling of urea between the collecting duct, interstitium and the ascending limb of loop of Henle. This recycling helps in the concentration of urine. For concentration of urine to be brought about a hyperosmotic medullary interstitium has to be maintained.
- Reabsorption occurs by a process of passive diffusion.

Concentration of urine

Concentration mechanism of urine: Depending on the body water content the volume of water excreted from the body in the form of urine can be altered. Because of the operation of the counter current systems in the kidney, the concentration of the urine can be brought about.

In the kidney there are two counter-current systems:

a. Counter-current multiplier contributed by the loop of Henle of the juxtamedullary nephrons

b. Counter-current exchanger contributed by the vasa recta.

There can be operation of these systems as counter-current systems, due the fact that they possess the following criteria:

- Flow in the two limbs will be in opposite direction to each other.
- Flow in the two limbs will be parallel to each other.

Operation of the counter-current system in these nephrons is because of the reason that there is a gradual increase in the osmolarity of the interstitium in the renal medulllary region reaching a peak of 1200 mOsm/L of water at the renal papilla due to the operation of the loop of Henle of juxtamedullary nephrons as counter-current

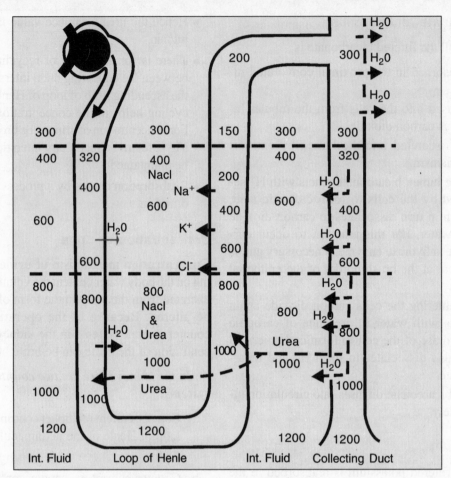

Fig 2.8 Counter-current multiplier

multiplier system. The loop of Henle of juxta-medullary nephrons are embedded in the hyper-osmotic interstitium and the length of these loops will be much when compared to the length of loop of Henle of cortical nephrons. The collecting ducts of all the nephrons pass through the medullary interstitium and contribute for concentration of urine by increasing water reabsorption.The water reabsorption at this part is due to action of anti diuretic hormone.

Counter-current multiplier (Fig. 2.8)

During the process of concentration of urine, when the filtrate passes through the descending limb of loop of Henle of juxtamedullary neph-rons, water keeps getting diffused from the tubule into the interstitium (along the osmotic gradient) which is hyperosmotic. This ensures the gradual increase in the osmolality of the tubular fluid reaching equilibrium with the surrouding inter-stitium, due to a relative increase in the concen-tration of osmotically active substances in the tubular fluid. Due to this a maximum of 1200 mOsm/L osmolality occurs in tubular fluid at the bend of the loop.

When the filtrate passes through the ascend-ing part of the loop now, the active co-transport of sodium, potassium and chloride into the interstitium gradually decreases the osmolality of the tubular fluid. The thick ascending limb of loop of Henle is impermeable to water. The osmolality of the filtrate reaching the beginning of distal convoluted tubules will be either hypo-/iso-osmotic. Finally when this filtrate passes through the collecting duct, due to the action of anti diuretic hormone, water keeps getting reabsorbed and the urine will attain a higher osmolality. In addition to facilitating water reabsorption, anti diuretic hormone will also help for urea to diffuse from the collecting duct into the interstitium which ultimately gets recycled as it diffuses from the interstitium to ascending limb of loop of Henle.

Counter-current exchanger (Fig. 2.9)

Much like the loop of Henle of juxtamedullary nephrons, which is embedded in the hyperosmotic interstitium in renal medulla, the vasa recta, which accompany the renal tubules of these nephrons, are also exposed to this hyperosmotic situation. Unlike the epithelial cells of renal tubules that are selectively permeable, the endothelial cells lining the vasa recta is freely permeable. Because of this when plasma flows through the descending limb of vasa recta, there will be slight influx of ions like sodium chloride and a simultaneous efflux of water into the interstitium. These processes ensure equilibration of osmolality of plasma with the interstitium. In the asceding limb the reversal of the events bring about a decrease of the osmolality of plasma. Finally the plasma leaving the vasa recta may have an osmolality of 325 mOsm/L as against a inflow plasma osmolality of 300 mOsm/L of water.

Secretion

Some of the substances are also secreted into the renal tubules at different parts. hydrogen ion is secreted at almost all the parts of the tubules whereas potassium is secreted at distal convoluted tubules. Some amount of creatinine also gets secreted and hence the creatinine clearance value is more than glormerular filtration rate.

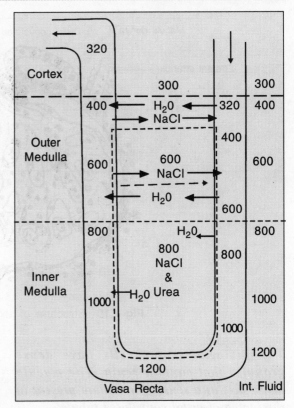

Fig 2.9 Counter-current exchanger

Diuretics are substances, which increase the urine output. Some of the commonly used diuretics are loop diuretics, spironolactone and acetazolamide. The loading of body with water can increase the urine output as well.

JUXTAGLOMERULAR APPARATUS

Juxtaglomerular apparatus (Fig. 2.10)

This is specialized structure in the kidney, which is composed of 3 different types of cells namely

- *Specialized smooth muscle cells of the arteriolar walls – juxtaglomerular cells.*
- *Specialized epithelial cells lining the distal convoluted tubules – macula densa.*
- *Between the above two there are certain other cells known as Lacis cells.*

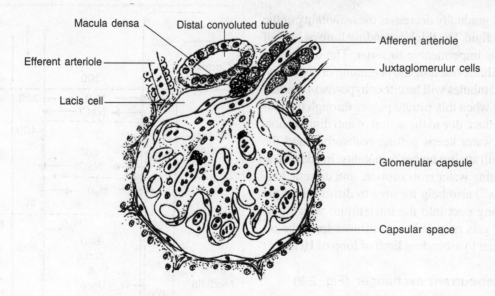

Fig 2.10 Structure of juxtaglomerular apparatus

The juxtaglomerular cells have dense granules that contain renin. The macula densa acts as a sensor for sodium present in the lumen of distal convoluted tubule.

The juxtaglomerular apparatus (JGA) is concerned with the operation of the renin angiotensin system. *Renin secreted by the juxta glomerular cells will act on angiotensinogen that is in circulation and converts it to angiotensin I. This further gets converted to angiotensin II by the action of the converting enzyme from the lungs. Some of the factors which influence renin secretion are: (a) decreased blood pressure or blood volume, (b) sympathetic nerve stimulation, and (c) decreased sodium in distal convoluted tubule. Angiotensin II exerts the actions on the different parts of body.*

The actions are

- *It acts on the smooth muscle of blood vessels and brings about the vasoconstriction and thereby help in the regulation of blood pressure.*

- *Helps to bring about the auto-regulation of the blood flow to the kidney.*
- *Stimulates the secretion of aldosterone hormone from the adrenal cortex.*
- *It also stimulates the thirst center.*

MICTURITION

Micturition is the periodic complete emptying of urinary bladder, which is normally under voluntary control in an adult.

The nerves supplying the bladder and urethra belong to the autonomic and somatic nervous system respectively. The autonomic nerves are the pelvic and hypogastric whereas the somatic nerve is the pudic/pudendal. The pelvic afferent carries the impulses from the stretch receptors present in the wall of the bladder and sympathetic afferent carries the pain impulses from the bladder.

At the time of voiding (micturition)

- *Pelvic afferent carries the impulses from the stretch receptors present in the wall of the bladder.*

- *Detrusor muscle, which is present in the wall of the bladder, gets the excitatory impulses through the pelvic nerve (S 2, 3 and 4) that is stimulated by the impulses coming along the pelvic afferent due to the stimulation of stretch receptors in the walls of the bladder.*

- *When the muscle is contracting the internal urethral sphincter relaxes and urine flows from the bladder into the urethra.*

- *Entry of urine into the urethra will stimulate the stretch receptors present in the posterior urethra.*

- *The somatic afferent nerve fibres (pudic) carry impulses from here.*

- *Somatic afferent impulses ultimately inhibit the efferent (pelvic) excitatory nerves (S 2, 3 and 4) supplying the external urethral sphincter (which is made up skeletal muscle).*

- *So the external urethral sphincter relaxes and the urine gets voided from the body* (Fig. 2.11).

There will be reinforcing impulses coming from the pontine centers to the spinal centers, which facilitate the complete voiding of the urine.

In the case of the adult the higher centers can regulate the activity of the primary centers of the spinal cord and hence it is under voluntary control. In infants in whom the higher control is yet to get established and hence the process of voiding is purely involuntary/reflex mechanism.

In the case of the adult after complete transection of spinal cord it can also become a purely a reflex during the stage of recovery of reflex activity due to the loss of higher center control over spinal centers present in the sacral segments of spinal cord (as seen in paraplegics).

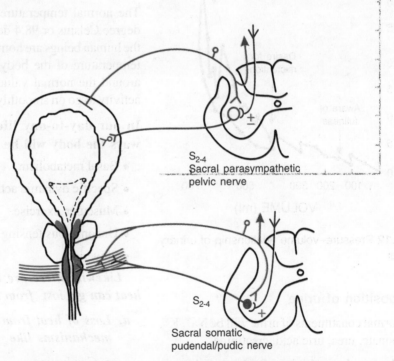

S₂₋₄
Sacral parasympathetic
pelvic nerve

S₂₋₄

Sacral somatic
pudendal/pudic nerve

Fig 2.11 Motor nerves involved in micturition

CYSTOMETROGRAM

Cystometrogram is graphical representation of the relationship between the volume of urine in bladder and the pressure in urinary bladder (Fig.2.12).

The configuration is due to plasticity property demonstrated by the smooth muscle present in the wall of the bladder and also because of the Laplace law, which is obeyed by the bladder. According to the law pressure developed in any spherical visceral structure is directly proportional to twice the tension (T) and inversely proportional to the radius (R).

$$P = \frac{2T}{R}$$

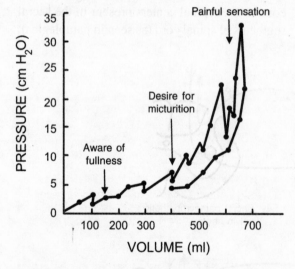

Fig 2 .12 Pressure–volume relationship of urinary bladder

Composition of urine

The normal constituents of urine will be Na^+, K^+, bicarbonate, urea, uric acid, creatinine.

- *Abnormal constituents of urine are* glucose, proteins, blood, bile salts.

- *In 24 hours sample of urine, specific gravity may range from 1005 to 1030 and urine of a normal person is slightly acidic most of the times.*

Anuria means there is no urine formation/excretion whereas in oliguria the volume of urine formed decreases considerably.

Renal failure

- Leads to the loss of function of kidney and hence the homeostasis of the body suffers.

- The person will not be able to survive if remedial measures are not employed.

- The measure may be temporary like the dialysis (haemodialysis or peritoneal) or permanent like the renal transplantation.

SKIN AND THERMOREGULATION

The normal temperature of body is around 37 degree Celsius or 98.4 degree Fahrenheit. Since the human beings are homoeothermic animals the temperature of the body should be maintained around the normal value for all the enzymatic activity to go on smoothly.

In our day-to-day life there are so many ways the body will be producing heat, like

- Basal metabolism
- Specific dynamic action of food
- Muscular exercise
- Unconscious tensing of muscles
- Shivering.

Likewise there are many ways by which heat can get lost from the body.

a. Loss of heat from the body by physical mechanisms like

- Conduction
- Convection

- Radiation
- Vaporization of water from the body (insensible perspiration).

b. *Increase in cutaneous blood flow to facilitate the heat loss by above processes.*

c. *Exposure of body surface area to increase radiation heat loss.*

d. *Vaporization of sweat.*

Thermoregulation

Mechanisms of heat gain/loss

- *Physical*
- *Physiological*
- *Behavioral*

For regulation of body temperature the centers are present in the hypothalamus and thermo receptors are present in the skin (peripheral) and in the hypothalamus (central). The peripheral thermo receptors sense the temperature of blood flowing the skin as well as the ambient temperature, whereas the central thermoreceptors sense the temperature of the blood flowing through the hypothalamus. When body wants to lose heat the heat loss mechanisms become more active and heat gain mechanisms are inhibited and vice versa happens when the body wants to gain heat.

In the hypothalamus there are heat gain and heat loss centers. The heat gain center is located in the posterior hypothalamus and heat loss center in the anterior hypothalamus. Apart from these two centers, there is also presence of biologic thermostat in the preoptic nucleus region of hypothalamus. A coordinated functioning of all these centers will help in the regulation of body temperature.

Efferent impulses from the hypothalamus through the sympathetic nerves reach the:

- Smooth muscle of blood vessels.
- Eccrine sweat glands present in the skin.
- Adrenal medulla to alter the secretion of the hormone catecholamines.

Apart from the role of nerves, there is alteration in the secretion of the hormones also during thermoregulation. The secretion of the hormones namely adrenaline, nor adrenaline (catecholamines) and thyroxin gets altered. These hormones increase the metabolic rate of the body and hence known as calorigenic hormones.

The most common condition in which the body temperature increases (pyrexia) is in fever. Any infectious state usually results in onset of fever. When body temperature is more than 104 degree Fahrenheit it is known as hyperpyrexia.

When body temperature is less than normal it is known as hypothermia. It can be accidental like accidents of ship on high seas, in temperate countries during the winter season when people do not have the proper shelter. In hospital set up hypothermia is induced during cardiac and neurosurgeries.

Skin

It is the outer most covering on the body. It performs many functions. Some of the important functions of the skin are:

- **Protection** –It acts as a mechanical barrier between the subcutaneous tissues and the surrounding environment and hence prevents the micro organisms invading the body.
- **Sense organ** –It has many types of receptors, which help us to perceive the sensations like touch, pressure, pain, temperature.

- **Thermoregulation** –It is due to its ability to transfer heat from one body to another along the thermal gradient by various physical and also by physiological mechanisms. The sweat glands present in the skin have a vital role to play. Alteration in the skin blood flow and opening of arteriovenous anastomosis as the situation demands will also take place during thermoregulation.

- **Secretory** – Apart from the sweat that is secreted by sweat glands there is secretion of sebum by sebaceous glands, which is responsible for the maintenance of the smooth texture of the skin.

- **Absorption** – Many of the lipid-based substances like creams, ointments get absorbed through the skin.

- **Excretory** – Some of the substances like salts, urea and fatty substances get excreted.

- **Endocrine** — Exposure of the skin to the light rays from the sun help for the endogenous production of vitamin D.

3

Gastrointestinal Tract

- Ingestion of food
- Secretion
- Digestion
- Absorption
- Excretion

Digestion can be of two types

- The mechanical breakdown of the foodstuff.
- The chemical breakdown by the action of the enzymes. The enzymes of the GI tract have the ability to act on almost all types of food like carbohydrate, fats and proteins.

INTRODUCTION

The structures present between the mouth and anus (both included) constitute the gastrointestinal system. Gastro intestinal tract has the following functions:

ORAL CAVITY

Not only helps for the ingestion of food but also brings about the mastication of food.

Mastication (chewing of food) helps

- Softening of the food
- Mechanical breakdown of food

- Mixing of saliva with the food
- Food to reach the body temperature.

The incisor teeth help for breaking, canines for tearing and molar and premolars for grinding the food. The movement of the jaws during the mastication is supported by the muscles of mastication namely temporalis, masseter, medial and lateral pterygoid. The upper jaw position is fixed and it is only the lower jaw that moves upwards, downwards and laterally. Mastication can be voluntary or involuntary depending on the situation. Muscles of cheek and tongue help to mix the food with the saliva so that the food gets crushed and there is formation of bolus.

SALIVARY GLANDS

These are the first glands we come across along the GI tract.

The group of salivary glands includes
- Parotid
- Submaxillary or submandibular
- Sublingual

The secretion from these glands reaches the oral cavity through special duct sys tem from the respective glands. Ebner's glands present in the tongue secrete lingual lipase.

The volume of saliva secreted per day is about 1000 ml.

The composition of saliva is
- 99% water
- Inorganic substances like Na^+, K^+, HCO^-_3, and Cl^-
- Organic substances like salivary amylase, lysozymes and mucus
- pH of saliva is about 6-7

The concentration of Na^+ in saliva depends on the rate of secretion . After saliva gets secreted from the acini when it passes through the ducts there is subsequent alteration in the composition. For every Na^+ that is taken back one K^+ is added on. Hence slower is the rate of secretion more is the content of K^+ in saliva.

Functions of saliva

- **Helps for perception of taste:** The food has to be made water soluble and then the chemical substances present in the food are able to stimulate the taste receptors present in the oral cavity.

- **Formation of bolus** is essential for the easy swallowing of the food. The water content of saliva and also the mucus aid this.

- **Digestive function** is because of the amylase present. This enzyme has the ability act on the cooked starch only. So the chemical digestion of food starts in the oral cavity.

- **Keeps the oral cavity moist:** This is essential for the proper articulation of speech.

- **Protective function** is aided by the presence of lysozymes, which have bactericidal function and hence destroy the micro-organisms that enter the oral cavity.

- **Excretory function** includes the excretion of some of the metals like lead, mercury.

- **Help to maintain the water balance** because when the body water content is reduced, rate of saliva secretion decreases and hence we feel the sensation of thirst.

Regulation of secretion

- It is brought about by a reflex mechanism.

- It is purely under the control of the nerves that belong to the autonomic nervous system.

The whole of GI tract movement and secretion is stimulated by the action of the parasympathetic nerves supplying it. Hence these nerves are known as the secretomotor nerves. Sympathetic nerve stimulation leads to the decrease in the motility and secretion in GI tract.

- ***The most important reflex to operate for the regulation of salivary secretion is called the unconditioned reflex.***

This reflex operates right from birth and there is no formal learning is necessary unlike for the conditioned reflex.

Unconditioned reflex

- Food in the oral cavity stimulates the taste receptors (within taste buds) present in the mouth.
- Afferent impulses are carried by facial (ant.

$2/3^{rd}$ of tongue), glossopharyngeal (post. $1/3^{rd}$ of tongue) and by the vagus nerve from the other parts of oral cavity to the CNS.

- These impulses reach the nucleus of tractus solitarius present in the brain stem.
- Impulses from this nucleus will reach the superior and inferior salivary nuclei, which are also present in the brain stem.
- Efferent impulses (Fig. 3.1) from the superior salivary nucleus reach submandibular and sublingual glands through facial nerve and from the inferior salivary nucleus reach the parotid glands through the glossopharyngeal nerve.

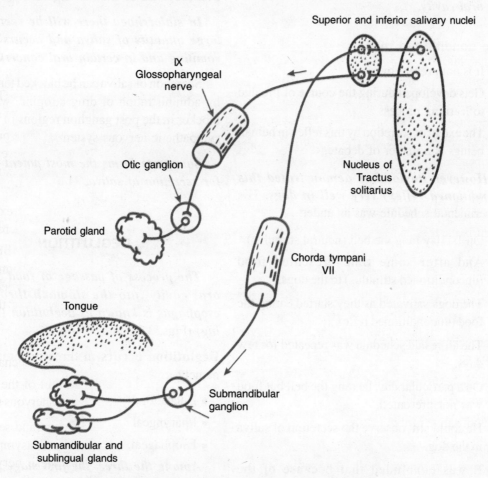

Fig 3.1 Parasympathetic innervation to salivary glands

- When the glands get stimulated there is secretion of saliva.

Apart from the stimulation of taste receptors, there will be stimulation of touch receptors in the oral cavity. From these receptors afferent impulses will be carried by the trigeminal nerve to salivary nuclei and other responses follow as explained above.

The neurotransmitter released from these parasympathetic nerve terminals is acetylcholine (ACh). The action of ACh at the post-ganglionic regions can be blocked by atropine and is popular method to decrease the rate of salivary secretion during any surgery involving oral cavity.

The conditioned reflex

- It is not present by birth.
- Gets developed during the course of life due to learning process.
- The extent of secretion by this reflex in human beings is a matter of debate.

However Pavlov has demonstrated this (conditioned reflex) very well in dogs. His experimental schedule was as under:

- On 1st day rang the bell (neutral stimulus).
- And after some time presented food (unconditioned stimulus) to the dogs.
- The dogs salivated as they started eating the food (unconditioned reflex).
- The aforesaid schedule was repeated for few days.
- On a particular day, he rang the bell but food was not presented.
- He could still observe the secretion of saliva in the dog.
- It was concluded that because of the association of bell sound preceding the food

presentation during the training period, the dog started secreting saliva in anticipation of the food.

This type of reflex, which develops due to learning process, is known as conditioned reflex and the stimulus (bell sound in this case) is the neutral stimulus to start with, later on gets converted to conditioned stimulus and the secretion of saliva that is observed for ringing of the bell alone is known as conditioned reflex.

Applied aspects

Xerostomia means scanty secretion of saliva (dryness of mouth) e.g. in anxiety.

In sialorrhoea there will be secretion of large quantity of saliva and occurs prior to vomiting and in certain oral cancers.

Secretion of saliva can be blocked temporarily by administration of drug atropine, which is a blocker in the post ganglion regions of the parasympathetic nervous system.

Sour taste forms the most potent stimulus for secretion of saliva.

DEGLUTITION

The process of passage of food from the oral cavity into the stomach through the esophagus is known as deglutition (swallowing) (Figs. 3.2 and 3.3).

Deglutition occurs in three different stages namely

- Buccal/oral
- Pharyngeal
- Esophageal.

Among the three, the first stage is voluntary and the rest are brought about reflexly.

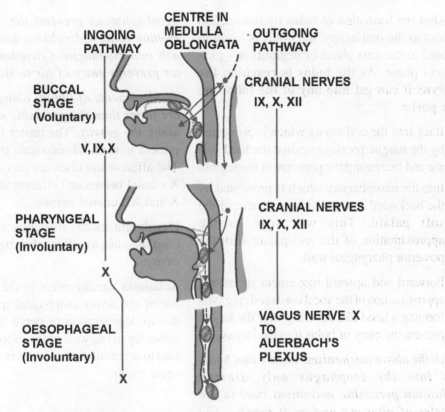

INGOING PATHWAY

CENTRE IN MEDULLA OBLONGATA

OUTGOING PATHWAY

CRANIAL NERVES IX, X, XII

BUCCAL STAGE (Voluntary)

V, IX, X

CRANIAL NERVES IX, X, XII

PHARYNGEAL STAGE (Involuntary)

X

OESOPHAGEAL STAGE (Involuntary)

X

VAGUS NERVE X TO AUERBACH'S PLEXUS

Fig 3.2 Stages in deglutition and nerves involved

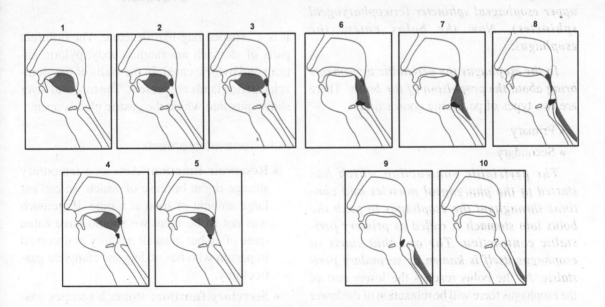

Fig 3.3 Passage of bolus during deglutition

After the formation of bolus by mastication process in the oral cavity, the bolus is ready to proceed to the next phase of deglutition – pharyngeal phase. **As the bolus is reaching the pharynx it can get into any of the following four parts:**

- Back into the oral cavity which is prevented by the tongue pressing against the hard palate and increasing the pressure in the region.

- Into the nasopharynx which is prevented by the backward and upward movement of the soft palate. This will lead to the approximation of the soft palate with the posterior pharyngeal wall.

- Forward and upward movement of larynx, approximation of the vocal cords and epiglottis forming a hood like covering over the larynx prevent the entry of bolus into the larynx.

All the above mechanisms ensure that bolus gets into the esophagus only. During deglutition peristaltic movement start in the muscles of pharynx and as it reaches the esophagus it leads to the relaxation of the upper esophageal sphincter (cricopharyngeal sphincter). Now the bolus enters the esophagus.

In the esophagus the peristaltic movements bring about the propulsion of the bolus. There are two types of peristaltic contractions

- Primary
- Secondary

The peristaltic contraction which has started in the pharyngeal muscles and continue throughout the esophagus to push the bolus into stomach is called as primary peristaltic contraction. The one that starts in esophagus itself is known as secondary peristalsis. As the bolus reaches the lower part of the esophagus there will be relaxation of the lower esophageal sphincter and bolus is pushed into the stomach. *The presence of the lower esoph-*

ageal sphincter prevents the reflux or regurgitation of the hydrochloric acid from the stomach into esophagus. Cricopharyngeal sphincter prevents entry of air to stomach.

Movements of liquids along the esophagus are faster than the peristaltic wave as it moves along the gravity. The center for deglutition is present in medulla oblongata in the brain stem. The afferent impulses are carried by V, IX and X cranial nerves and efferent are carried by IX, X and XII cranial nerves.

Dysphagia means difficulty to swallow seen conditions like tonsillitis, pharyngitis, ulcers in oral cavity.

Achalasia cardia refers to the congenital failure of the lower esophageal sphincter to relax due to degeneration of nerve fibres around the sphincter in the wall of the esophagus. This will lead to accumulation of bolus in the lower esophageal region.

STOMACH

It is 'C' shaped bag-like structure. The different parts of stomach are fundus, body, pyloric antrum and pyloric canal. In the walls of the stomach gastric glands are present. The mucosal layer shows pits into which the gastric glands open.

Functions of stomach

- **Reservoir function:** Acts as a temporary storage organ because of which we can eat large amount of food at a time. If stomach was not to be there we should have eaten quite often but in small quantity as observed in person who has undergone complete gastrectomy.

- **Secretory function:** stomach secretes gastric juice (HCl, pepsin), which has important role to play in digestion of food.

- **Propulsion of food:** There is delivery of small quantity of food properly mixed with gastric secretion into the small intestine for a thorough digestion and absorption.
- **Protective function** is contributed by the high acidity in the stomach by HCl, which has bactericidal action.
- **Haemopoietic function** is due to secretion of intrinsic factor secreted by stomach. Intrinsic factor is very much essential for the absorption of vitamin B_{12} and the acidic medium is necessary for conversion of ferric iron to ferrous iron before absorption.
- **It also helps in expulsion of some of the harmful substances like poisons by initiating a process called vomiting.**
- **Endocrine function** is because of the secretion of the hormone gastrin that also stimulates the secretion of gastric juice.
- **Absorptive function:** Substances like water and alcohol get absorbed in the stomach itself.

Gastric juice

Volume secreted per day 1000 ml.

- pH 1.2 – 2.0
- Inorganic substances Na^+, K^+, H^+, Cl^- (HCl)
- Organic substances are pepsinogen, intrinsic factor, mucus etc.

HCl is secreted by the parietal or oxyntic cells which also secretes intrinsic factor. Peptic or chief cells secrete pepsinogen and the neck cells secrete mucus (Fig. 3.4). Gastrin hormone is secreted into the circulation by the G cells present in the pyloric antrum region.

Mechanism of secretion of HCl

- Ionization of water leads to the formation of H^+ and OH^- inside the parietal cell.
- CO_2 reacts with H_2O and H_2CO_3 is formed.
- Dissociation of carbonic acid leads to the formation of HCO_3^- and H^+.

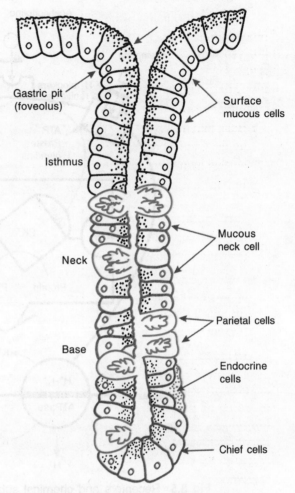

Fig 3.4 Cell types in gastric glands

- H^+ reacts with OH^- to form one more molecule of water.
- H^+, which got ionized from H_2O, will get pumped into the canaliculi in exchange for the K^+.
- HCO_3^- ion produced in the cell enters the blood stream in exchange for the Cl^-. The Cl^- also gets pumped into the canaliculi.
- The reaction between the hydrogen and chloride ions occurs in the canaliculi and result in formation of HCl.

Histaminergic (H_2 receptors), cholinergic

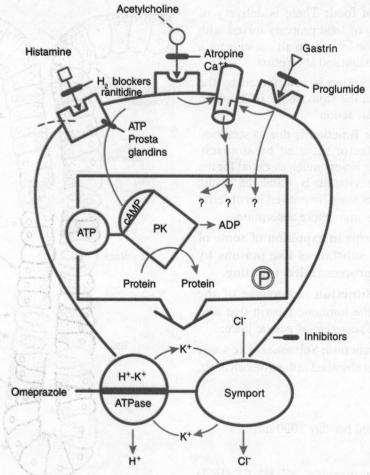

Fig 3.5 Receptors and chemical substances acting on the parietal cells

and gastrin receptors are found on the parietal cells (Fig. 3.5).

Drugs like

- Ranitidine
- Cimetidine
- Famotidine

block histaminergic receptors activity.

- Cholinergic receptors can be blocked by atropine.
- Gastrin receptors can be blocked by proglumide.

In addition to the above, the activity of proton pump (K^+- H^+ pump) of the canaliculi can be inhibited by the action of pump inhibitors like omeprazole, useful in the treatment of peptic ulcers.

Many of these are drugs of choice in treatment of peptic ulcers.

Regulation of secretion of gastric juice

1. Cephalic phase (psychic phase)
2. Gastric phase
3. Intestinal phase.

Cephalic phase

During this phase the afferent impulses coming from the head region (structures present above the stomach) of the body will stimulate the secretion. In this phase even before the food enters the stomach there is stimulation for the gastric juice secretion (about 30% secretion is because of this phase). *This phase is influenced by the neural mechanism and the efferent nerve involved is vagus.*

Mechanism of operation of this phase is

- Food in the mouth.
- Taste receptors get stimulated.
- Afferent impulses from the taste receptors are carried by the VII, IX and X cranial nerves to the brain stem.
- These impulses on reaching the brain stem stimulate the dorsal motor nucleus of X.
- The efferent impulses will be carried by the X cranial nerve from the nucleus to the gastric glands.
- Gastric glands get stimulated.
- There will be secretion of the gastric juice.

Impulses coming from cerebral cortex or hypothalamus can also influence the activity of the dorsal motor nucleus of vagus present in the brain stem and thereby alter the secretion of gastric juice.. This phase prepares the stomach for the reception of the bolus for further digestion without any time delay. Apart from the taste receptor stimulation, the sight of food, thought of food can also stimulate the secretion.

Pavlov first demonstrated cephalic phase of gastric juice secretion in dogs.

- The esophagus of the dog was cut and the two cut ends were brought to the anterior surface of the neck.

- When the dog was given food, the dog relished eating food but food did not reach the stomach, as the continuity of the esophagus had been lost.
- Food came out of the upper cut end of the esophagus.
- But Pavlov still observed by aspirating the contents of the stomach, that there was secretion of the gastric juice.
- After bilateral vagotomy there was abolition of the secretion when the experiment was repeated.

Hence he concluded that cephalic phase of gastric juice secretion is mediated by the efferent vagus nerve only. This experiment is known as Sham feeding (false feeding). Sham feeding like situation can be imitated in human beings also. *Esophagotomy is not advisable but ask the person to chew food and spit out and thereby mimic the sham-feeding situation.*

Gastric phase

- This is the most important phase (50% secretion is because of this phase).
- In this phase the volume of gastric juice secreted is high and duration of secretion is also more prolonged.
- There should be presence of food in stomach or a mere distension of the wall of the stomach is essential for this phase.
- It is mediated by both the neural (X nerve) and hormonal (gastrin) mechanisms.
- The two different mechanisms potentiate the action of each other and hence when both the mechanisms are acting it leads to a copious secretion of gastric juice.
- About 1/2 of the total volume of gastric juice secreted is due to this phase.

Neural mechanism is brought about by both the short and long loops. Distension of the wall of the stomach stimulates a variety of receptors in the wall of the stomach. Afferent impulses are carried by vagal fibres, which will have a collateral. These collateral end on the intrinsic nerve plexus (Meissner's plexus) present in the submucosal region and stimulate them. These intrinsic plexus ultimately stimulate the glands to secrete gastric juice. *Since the whole activity is happening within the structures present in the wall of the stomach and without involving the central nervous system, this is known as the short loop mechanism.*

Long loop mechanism (Vagovagal reflex) is where the afferent vagal fibres carry the impulses to the brain stem from the receptors in the wall of the stomach. These fibres stimulate the dorsal motor nucleus present in the brain stem, which in turn sends efferent impulses along the vagal efferent to gastric glands. The gastric glands get stimulated and there will be secretion of gastric juice. *This is known as vagovagal reflex as vagus nerve is involved both in the afferent and efferent limbs of the reflex activity.*

Neural mechanism of gastric juice secretion can be demonstrated by the construction of *Pavlov's pouch, which is vagally innervated pouch and there will be a copius secretion of gastric juice in this pouch (because both neural and hormonal influence will be there in this pouch).*

When partially digested food enters the stomach especially the antral region, the distension of the antrum stimulates the secretion of the gastrin hormone from the G cells. Gastrin enters the circulation and on reaching the gastric glands stimulates the secretion of gastric juice.

The role of this hormone in gastric phase of gastric juice secretion can be demonstrated by construction of Heidenhain's pouch that is vagally denervated. When compared to Pavlov's pouch in Heidenhain's pouch the volume of gastric juice secreted is very less, as only hormonal mechanism is operating.

Factors influencing gastrin release are:

- Luminal factors like peptides, amino acids and distension of stomach.
- Neural factors like vagal stimulation.
- Gastrin secretion is inhibited by secretin, GIP, VIP, acid pH.

Intestinal phase

As the food enters the duodenum, the influence from the intestine on the functioning of the stomach is mostly inhibitory to ensure a proper digestion, absorption and to prevent the ulcer formation at the duodenum region. The inhibitory influence not only affects secretion but also the motility of the stomach. The hormones secreted by the intestine bring about most of the inhibition.

The hormones involved are secretin and cholecystokinin-pancreozymin (CCK-PZ). Hormones secreted from the intestinal region enter circulation and act on stomach to reduce secretion and motility. Apart from this, the neural mechanism also has a role, which is known as enterogastric reflex. Even this reflex is an example for vago vagal reflex as both in the afferent and efferent pathway the nerve involved is vagus.

Motor (motility) functions of stomach: Stomach exhibits three motor functions namely

- Receptive relaxation
- Movement of stomach to facilitate the mixing of food
- Gastric emptying for propulsion of chyme into the intestine.

Apart from these, in certain situation it can also initiate the process of vomiting.

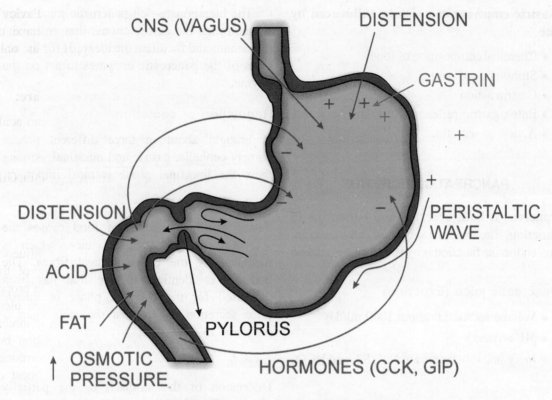

Fig 3.6 Factors influencing gastric motility

Receptive relaxation

Due to the aforesaid movement it exhibits, stomach can also act as a temporary storage organ. When food enters the stomach, the muscles in the body of the stomach get relaxed. This prevents the build up of tension in the wall and the smooth muscle which is present in the wall of the stomach demonstrates the property of plasticity. Without the receptive relaxation, intake of large quantity of food in one go is not possible.

Mixing of food

It begins at the middle part of the stomach. Mild peristaltic wave begin here at the rate of 3/minute and move toward the antrum. This causes the mixing of food with the secretions of gastric glands.

Propulsion of food

As the pyloric sphincter opening is narrow, a large part of food is unable to pass through this region to reach the small intestine during the strong peristaltic contractions. A small portion of the food is made to pass through the pyloric region into the duodenum and a major part is reverted into the body of the stomach and this is known as retropulsion. This facilitates mixing of the food as well.

Factors influencing gastric emptying (Fig. 3.6)

- Nature of food (physical and or chemical)
- Osmolarity of food
- Extent of distension of the stomach
- Acidity in the duodenum.

Gastric emptying can also be influenced by the

- Chemical composition of food
- Stimulation of nerves
- Gastrin action
- Enterogastric reflexes
- Action of secretin.

PANCREATIC SECRETION

Pancreas is both exocrine and endocrine in function. The exocrine secretion is by the acini and endocrine function is by islets of Langerhans.

Pancreatic juice (Exocrine)

- Volume secreted is about 1000 ml/day
- pH around 8
- Inorganic substances are Na^+, K^+, and HCO_3
.

Organic constituents (enzymes) are:

- Amylolytic – pancreatic amylase
- Lipolytic – pancreatic lipase, co-lipase
- Proteolytic- trypsin, chymotrypsin, carboxypeptidase A & B etc.
- Nucleolytic– ribo-and deoxyribonucleases

Most of the enzymes are secreted in the inactive form, otherwise there can be auto digestion of the pancreatic tissue. The enzyme that get activated by the intestinal secretions is trypsinogen. This activation is by action of enterokinase (enteropeptidase) and converts trypsinogen to trypsin.

This trypsin can further bring about the activation of more amount of trypsinogen. This reaction is one of the examples of an autocatalytic reaction. Trypsin activates chymotrypsinogen, pro carboxy peptidase as well.

The bicarbonate-rich pancreatic juice helps to neutralize the acidic chyme that enters the duodenum and facilitate the ideal pH for the actions of the pancreatic enzymes to act on the chyme.

Regulation of secretion

Is brought about in three different phases namely cephalic, gastric and intestinal. Among these the intestinal phase is most important.

Cephalic phase

Taste, smell or thought of food causes the secretion of the pancreatic juice, which is mediated by the efferent vagal fibres. The pathway is identical to one that has been discussed for the cephalic phase of gastric juice secretion except that the end organ is pancreas in this case.

Gastric phase

Distension of the stomach or the partially digested food in the stomach stimulates the G cells to secrete gastrin. This gastrin enters the circulation and on reaching the pancreas stimulates secretion from the acini.

The neural influence from the stomach can also stimulate the secretion of pancreatic juice by vago vagal reflex.

Though there is influence from oral cavity and stomach with respect to pancreatic secretion, it is not very much.

Intestinal phase

As stated already this is the most important phase. Most of the regulation during this phase is mediated by the hormones namely secretin and cholecystokinin pancreozymin (CCK-PZ) secreted by the mucosal lining of the duodenum.

The neural influence from the small intestine on pancreatic juice secretion is by the vagovagal reflex but is not so important.

Hormonal influence on pancreatic secretion		
	Secretin	**CCK-PZ**
Site of secretion	Duodenum and jejunum	Duodenum and jejunum
Stimulus	Acid chyme	Chyme rich (duodenum) in fats and proteins.
Site of action	on ducts	on acini
Type of secretion	rich in HCO$_3$	rich in enzymes
Purpose served	Neutralizing the chyme	Digestion of food
Volume secreted	Large	Moderate

Acute pancreatitis

It is due to obstruction of the pancreatic ducts. This causes the digestion of the pancreatic tissue itself. In carcinoma of pancreas mostly the lipid digestion suffers. Protein digestion is partially affected and carbohydrate digestion doesn't get affected at all.

LIVER AND BILE

The bile secreted by the hepatocytes in the liver enters the gall bladder through the cystic duct and gets stored. During the storage time there will be certain alterations in the volume and composition of the bile in the gall bladder. The contractions of the gall bladder will empty the bile into the intestine through the bile duct.

Functions of liver

- Secretion of bile by the hepatocytes into the biliary canaliculi.
- Storage of glycogen and vitamin B$_{12}$, A and D. It also stores iron.

- Synthesis of almost all the plasma proteins except gamma globulin.
- Excretion of cholesterol and bile pigments.
- Haemopoietic function in fetal life
- Detoxification of certain hormones and drugs
- Reticuloendothelial function by the Kupffer's cells

Composition of bile

- Water 97%
- Bile salts – sodium and potassium taurocholates and glycocholates
- Bile pigment – bilirubin
- Cholesterol
- Inorganic salts
- Fatty acids
- Alkaline phosphatase
- Lecithin

Secretion of bile is continuous one whereas the emptying of bile into the intestine is intermittent. Bile secreted from the hepatocytes reach the gall bladder and get stored. In the gall bladder there is reabsorption of water and hence the volume of bile is reduced from the initial 2000 ml/day to about 500 ml/day that is reaching the intestine. While it is stored in the gall bladder bile becomes a little more acidic due to the absorption of HCO$_3$ ions and walls of the gall bladder also secrete mucus. **All these aspects constitute the** functions of the gall bladder.

Functions of the gall bladder are:

1. Storage of bile.
2. Concentration of bile.
3. Expulsion of bile.
4. Acidification of bile.

Bile salts are secreted by hepatocytes and they are

1. Sodium glycocholate and taurocholate

2. Potassium glycocholate and taurocholate.

Functions of bile salts

- **Emulsification of fats** is brought about by decreasing the surface tension. TAG (Triacyl glycerol) can easily break down to small units so that lipolytic enzymes can act on it.

- **Hydrotropic action:** Micelle formation allows fat to be made water-soluble and hence help for absorption of fats and fat-soluble vitamins through the enterocytes into the lacteals.

- **Keeps the cholesterol in solution:** This prevents the formation of gall stones.

- **Bactericidal action:** Bile salts do have some amount of bactericidal action and kill the bacteria in the intestinal regions.

Emptying of bile

This is brought about by the entry of chyme into the intestine. Presence of chyme in the intestine brings about the secretion of CCK-PZ from the mucosal lining of duodenum and jejunum. It reaches the gall bladder along the circulation and brings about the contraction of the smooth muscle present in the wall of the gall bladder and at the same time relaxes the sphincter of Oddi. *Any substance, which stimulates the release of bile from the gall bladder, is known as cholegogue and example is CCK-PZ.*

Choleretics: *There are substances which stimulate the secretion of bile from the hepatocytes of liver e.g. secretin, bile salts themselves and also CCK-PZ.* About 98% of the bile salts reaching the intestine are getting reabsorbed and hence get resecreted. Most of the reabsorption occurs in the terminal parts of ileum and they get into entero hepatic circulation for getting resecreted from the liver.

Cholecystography: *It is the radiographic study of the gall bladder function.* The study requires administration of some radio opaque substance through the oral route. (If the radio opaque substance is given through the intravenous route to observe the bile duct, it is known as cholangiography).

The substance given through any of the above routes reach the liver, get secreted into the hepatic ducts along with the bile and thereby helps for radiographic study of the biliary tract. Deposition of the cholesterol in gall bladder/in the biliary tract leads to the formation of gall stones and this can be made out by the aforesaid studies.

SMALL INTESTINE

- The brush border of the epithelial (enterocytes) cells lining the small intestine release the enzymes into the lumen of the small intestine. The life span of enterocytes is about 3 days and as the cells are sloughed into the intestine, the lysis of the cells brings about the release of the enzymes into the lumen of the intestine.

- Most of the digestion and absorption occurs in duodenum and jejunum regions.

- Mucus from the Brunner's glands protects the duodenal wall from the acid of the stomach that has reached the intestine.

The enzymes released from the brush borders are:

- Amylolytic like sucrase, maltase and lactase.

- Proteolytic like dipeptidase, enteropeptidase, aminopeptidase.

- Lipolytic like intestinal lipase.

DIGESTION AND ABSORPTION

Carbohydrates

Polysaccharides like starch, disaccharides like sucrose, lactose are digested.

Salivary amylase acts on cooked starch and end products are maltotriose, maltose etc. In the small intestine

$$\text{Maltose} \xrightarrow{\text{Maltase}} \text{glucose + glucose}$$

$$\text{Sucrose} \xrightarrow{\text{Sucrase}} \text{glucose + fructose}$$

$$\text{Lactose} \xrightarrow{\text{Lactase}} \text{glucose + galactose}$$

Digestion of disaccharides occurs only in the mucosal epithelium. Carbohydrates are absorbed in the monosaccharide form into the capillaries of the villi of the small intestine. Most of the these monosaccharides are absorbed by a process of secondary active transport with the involvement of carrier protein much like what is observed in the kidneys.

Proteins

The digestion gets initiated in the stomach due to the action of the enzyme pepsin secreted by the chief cells. It acts on proteins to bring about the formation of oligopeptides.

In the small intestine there are many proteolytic enzymes coming from different parts, which ensure the complete digestion of proteins. The end products of protein digestion namely amino acids are absorbed into the blood vessels by a process of cotransport mechanism. In infants the intact proteins can get absorbed directly without any chemical break down e.g. colostrums, which contain maternal antibodies.

Fat digestion

Fat has to be made water-soluble by the formation of micelles. The emulsification action of the bile salts helps for the complete action of the lipolytic enzymes on fats. Triacyl glycerol is digested by the action of pancreatic lipase and colipase to form monuglycerides and free fatty acids. **The bile salts also help for the formation of mixed micelles which is essential for the absorption of fats and fat soluble vitamins. Enterocytes are impermeable to fats and fat-soluble vitamins without the micellar formation.** *Fatty acids and monglycerides will be passed on into the lacteals through the enterocytes.*

Absorption of water and minerals (Fig. 3.7)

Water gets absorbed almost throughout the

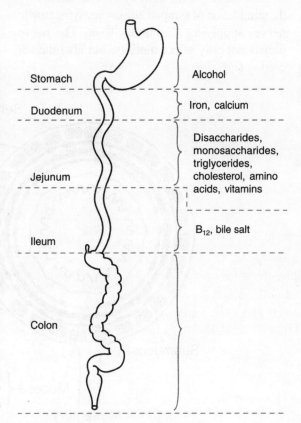

Fig 3.7 Absorption of substances in different parts of GI tract

Stomach — Alcohol

Duodenum — Iron, calcium

Jejunum — Disaccharides, monosaccharides, triglycerides, cholesterol, amino acids, vitamins

Ileum — B_{12}, bile salt

Colon

tract. Vitamin B_{12} and bile salts get absorbed in terminal part of ileum.

MOTILITY OF SMALL INTESTINE

Motility is because of the smooth muscles present in the wall of the small intestine. There are two types of muscles namely longitudinal bundle which is outer and inner will be the circular muscle layer. The activity of these muscles will be very much dependent on the nerve plexus present in the wall itself. These nerve plexuses (enteric nervous system) are called as myenteric/Auerbach and Meissner/submucosal.

The nerve plexus activity can be altered by the stimulation of sympathetic or parasympathetic nerves supplying alimentary tract. The nerve plexus not only affect motility, but also the secretion (Fig. 3.8).

Types of movements are (Fig. 3.9)

- Mixing type – segmentation.
- Propulsive / translatory type – peristalsis.

Segmentation: Small parts of intestine undergoes a series of contractions and dilations (relaxation) alternating. After some time the places where contraction occurred earlier, now dilates and earlier dilated part now contracts. This type of movement helps for mixing chyme with the digestive juices and also to bring new surface of the chyme to get exposed to the mucosal lining of intestine for better absorption.

Peristaltic movements occur throughout the length of the gastrointestinal tract. The first part where it appears is in the muscles of pharynx. The peristaltic movement is termed as propulsive or translatory movement.

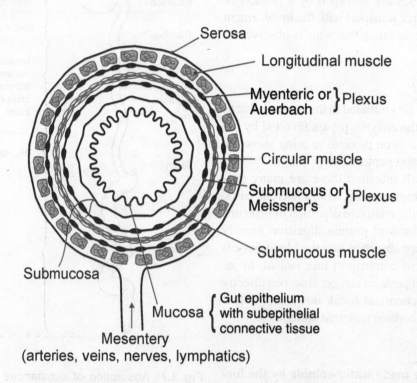

Fig 3.8 Transverse section of small intestine

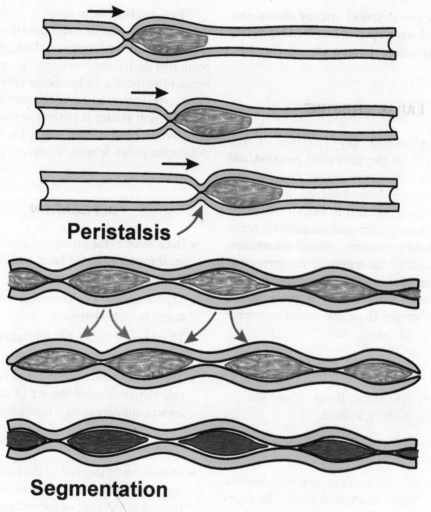

Peristalsis

Segmentation

Fig 3.9 Movements of small intestine

Peristaltic movements are responsible for the movements of chyme along the intestine. Presence of chyme in the intestine, distends the part of the intestine. This distension acts as a mechanical stimulus to the smooth muscle of the intestine. So just behind the place where the chyme is present a wave of constriction appears and in front of the chyme there will be receptive relaxation. A series of such contraction and relaxation move from the oral to the aboral end (as per the Starling's law of intestine/law of the gut) and help for the propulsion of the chyme.

Rate of segmentation movements in different parts of the intestine will be

- Duodenum — 10-12/min
- Jejunum — 6-10/min
- Ileum — 6-8/min.

The movements are affected by the activity of myenteric plexus (intrinsic). Parasympathetic nerve stimulation enhances the motility unlike the sympathetic that inhibits. Even in the absence of extrinsic nerves intestine demonstrates the movements.

Villi have two different types of movements namely the shortening and lengthening movement and whiplash movement.

LARGE INTESTINE

It does not secrete any enzymes. Large intestine begins at the ileocaecal junction and ends in anus. We come across haustrations/ puckerings in the large intestine due to the presence of tenia coli that is thrown into three longitudinal bands. The parasympathetic nerve supplies the large intestine. Vagal innervation extends upto $2/3^{rd}$ the length of the transverse colon. The remaining of the large intestine, the parasympathetic nerve supply is pelvic nerve which takes origin from the sacral segments ($S_{2, 3 \text{ and } 4}$) of spinal cord.

Functions of large intestine

1. Absorptive function: Brings about the absorption of water, sodium.

2. Temporary storage organ for feces and excretion of fecal matter.

3. Secretion of substances like bicarbonate, mucus. Water absorption makes the feces harder and the mucus helps for the fecal matter to remain bound to each other as a mass and the smooth passage of the same through rectum and anal canal.

4. Synthesis of certain vitamins (certain vitamins of B complex group and vitamin K) by the bacterial flora that is housed in the large intestine.

In the large intestine movements do occur. The different movements are

Segmentation, which is almost like, that is seen in the small intestine and helps for the mixing of the contents (mainly the undigested food) with that of the secretions of the large intestine.

Mass peristalsis is entirely different from the peristalsis seen in small intestine. It occurs around the time of defecation. Instead of a small portion of the intestine undergoing contraction, a series of peristaltic rushes occur rapidly involving a considerable length of the intestine. Due to this the fecal matter is pushed towards the rectum. When fecal matter enters the rectum the defecation reflex is brought about.

DEFECATION

- Defecation is the process of emptying of the fecal matter from the large intestine through the anal canal and anus.

- The frequency of defecation in any individual depends on his habits.

- The primary center for defecation is present in spinal cord (sacral segments).

- The higher center is present in cerebral cortex. Hence in adult the act of defecation is under voluntary control like micturition.

Mechanism of defecation

- Distension of the wall of the rectum leads to the stimulation of the mechanoreceptors present in the wall of the rectum.

- Pelvic fibres carry afferent impulses.

- On reaching the spinal cord they stimulate the motor neurons present in sacral segments.

- Efferent impulses come along the pelvic nerve ($S_{2, 3 \text{ and } 4}$) and stimulate the contraction of the smooth muscle present in the wall of the rectum and relaxation of the internal anal sphincter.

- Now the fecal matter gets pushed into the anal canal.

- In the anal canal there will be stimulation of the mechanoreceptors and the pudic nerve fibres carry afferent impulses and the impulses on reaching the sacral segments bring about the inhibition of the efferent pudic/pudendal nerve ($S_{2, 3 \text{ and } 4}$) supplying the external anal sphincter.

- The external anal sphincter relaxes and fecal matter is excreted.

Irritation of the large intestine causes less water to be absorbed and fecal matter rushes through the colon leading to diarrhea. When a person experiencess difficulty to bring about the process of defecation it is known as constipation.

VOMITING

Is the process by which the contents of the upper parts of the GI tract are thrown out of the body through the oral cavity. It is brought about by a reflex mechanism and the center is present in the floor of the fourth ventricle in medulla oblongata. Certain drugs like morphine, apomorphine can stimulate this area and initiate the process of vomiting.

When vomiting starts
- There will be increased salivation and sensation of nausea.
- Reverse peristalsis brings the regurgitation of food from the upper part of small intestine into the stomach.
- The closure of the glottis ensures that vomitus will not enter the larynx and trachea.
- The breath is held and the muscles of the abdominal wall contract raising the intra abdominal pressure.
- The lower esophageal sphincter relaxes and gastric contents are ejected out. Afferent impulses for the process of vomiting may also come from the upper part of small intestine, vestibular nuclei etc.

4

Endocrinology

- Introduction
- Thyroid gland
- Calcium metabolism
- Adrenal cortex and medulla
- Endocrine pancreas
- Anterior pituitary gland
- Posterior pituitary gland.

The hormonal functions in the body are
(Table 4.1)

- Regulation of the metabolism
- Regulation of water and electrolyte content
- Help for growth
- Also necessary for the reproduction
- In certain situations they help the body to withstand the stressful conditions.

INTRODUCTION

The study of hormones secreted by special glands that are ductless is known as endocrinology. Hormones are special chemical substances present constantly in circulation. The organ/tissue on which the hormone acts is known as target organ. The hormones carry chemical messages to almost all the parts of the body and hence are also important for regulation of functions of the body along with nervous system.

Table 4.1 General functions of hormones in the body

I. Growth	Development/Maturation
II. Regulate	Metabolism of Carbohydrate, Fat, Proteins Electrolytes, Water
III. Reproduction	Sexual function

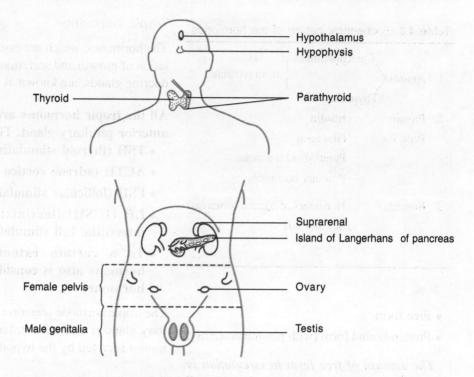

Fig 4.1 Location of endocrine organs in different parts of body

The endocrine glands are present in different parts of body (Fig. 4.1 & Table 4.2). Few of them are paired like adrenals and the others are un-paired like pituitary.

Table 4.2 List of endocrine glands

I.　Hypothalamus

II　Anterior and posterior pituitary

III.　Islets of Langerhans

IV.　Adrenal cortex and adrenal medulla

V.　Thyroid

VI.　Parathyroid

VII.　Testes/Ovaries

Essential endocrine glands

Which means that without the secretions of these glands the person can't survive.

The essential endocrine glands in the body are

- Parathyroid
- Adrenal cortex

Chemical nature (Table 4.3)

The biochemical nature of the hormone can be

- Peptide/ protein
- Steroid
- Amines

Peptide hormones can never be given orally as they get digested in the intestine.

Transport

Hormones are circulated in blood stream in two forms:

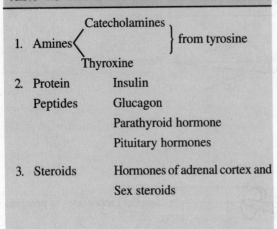

Table 4.3 Biochemical nature of the hormones

1. Amines	Catecholamines	from tyrosine
	Thyroxine	
2. Protein	Insulin	
Peptides	Glucagon	
	Parathyroid hormone	
	Pituitary hormones	
3. Steroids	Hormones of adrenal cortex and Sex steroids	

- Free form
- Protein-bound form (with plasma proteins).

The amount of free form in circulation is very less but still is important as it exerts all the biological actions of the hormone. The protein-bound form acts as a reservoir and gets released into free form as and when required. Apart from this the protein bound form can't get filtered in the kidneys and hence hormones loss from the body is minimised.

Degradation of hormones (Table 4.4)

Most of the hormones get metabolized in the target organs. Hormones belonging to steroid group get metabolized in the liver.

Table 4.4 Inactivation of hormones

1. By the target tissue
2. By the Liver/Kidney
   Conjugated either by glucuronyl transferase system or by SO_4

Tropic hormone

The hormones, which are essential for the regulation of growth and secretion of some other endocrine glands, are known as tropic hormones.

All the tropic hormones are secreted by the anterior pituitary gland. They are
- **TSH (thyroid stimulating hormone)**
- **ACTH (adreno cortico tropic hormone)**
- **FSH (follicular stimulating hormone)**
- **LH (ICSH) (leutinizing hormone or interstitial cell stimulating hormone)**
- **To a certain extent even growth hormone also is considered as a tropic hormone.**

The tropic hormone secretion from anterior pituitary gland is under the influence of neuro hormones secreted by the hypothalamus.

Mechanism of action

Second Messengers :	
Peptides and Catecholamines	↑Formation of - Cyclic AMP - Calcium - Phospholipid

Proteins and peptide hormones can bind to the cell membrane receptors. Hence when they act on the receptors, in the intracellular fluid part there will be alteration in the concentration of substances like cAMP, Ca^{++} or inositol triphosphate. These substances act as second messengers and exert all actions of the hormone in the intra cellular fluid region.

Steroid hormones can enter the cell through the cell membrane and bind to the receptors present in the cytoplasm or the nucleus. This increases the formation of mRNA and helps for synthesizing new proteins.

Estimation of hormones

Can be done by

- Radio immuno assay
- Spectrophotometer methods
- Bioassay.

How to establish the function or actions of hormones in the body? (Table 4.5)

Table 4.5 List of ways to establish hormonal actions in the body
1. Remove the suspected tissue and look for signs and symptoms
2. Prepare an extract - inject
3. Inject extract in larger amounts
4. Correlate with clinical conditions
5. Biochemical nature
6. Synthesis

Regulation of secretion of hormones can be brought about by different ways.

- **Feedback control** – wherein the concentration of the hormone in circulation can regulate its own secretion by acting through the hypothalamus or pituitary or both. The feed back control may be negative or positive. **In negative feed back, increase in the free form of hormone in circulation leads to decrease secretion of the same hormone, whereas in positive feedback it is vice versa by acting through the hypothalamus or anterior pituitary gland or both. Negative feed back control E.g. Thyroxin (refer regulation of secretion).**

- **Concentration of substances in plasma:** Concentration of substance in plasma can directly act on the endocrine glands and the secretion rate may be altered. E.g. the blood glucose level regulates insulin secretion.

(More is blood glucose, more will be secretion of insulin)

- **Neural influences:** The activity of the nervous system can also regulate the secretion of some hormones. *e.g.* Catecholamines secretion is regulated by sympathetic nerve activity. The neuroendocrine reflex can also be included here (for details refer oxytocin secretion).

- **Diurnal variation:** During 24 hours of the day, the rate of hormone secretion varies depending on the time. *e.g.* Secretion of ADH is more in the night than during day time. Even cortisol secretion has diurnal variation.

THYROID GLAND

The only superficial endocrine gland, the enlargement of which can be made out very easily. **The hormones secreted by this gland are**

- Thyroxine. (T_4)
- Triiodothyronine (T_3)
- Thyrocalcitonin (Calcitonin)

Among the three hormones, the follicular cells of the gland secrete the first two hormones (T_3 & T_4) and the last one (thyrocalcitonin) is by the para follicular cells. T_4 is also known as tetraiodothyronin and gets converted to T_3 at the time of action in the target organ. Calcitonin hormone will be disscussed along with calcium metabolism.

The steps in the biosynthesis of the hormone are

- **Iodide trapping** that is the uptake of iodine by the follicular cells from the plasma against the electrochemical gradient. The hormone

TSH secreted by the anterior pituitary gland affects this step. Substances like thiocyanate and perchlorate that are examples of antithyroid drugs can inhibit iodide trapping.

- **Oxidation of iodine:** Occurs inside the follicular cells by the action of the enzyme peroxidase. Drugs like thiouracil and carbimazole can inhibit this step and act as antithyroid drugs.
- **Organification:** Iodine gets incorporated to tyrosine amino acid present in the colloid and leads to the formation of MIT (Mono iodo tyrosine). On further iodination of MIT, there is formation of DIT (Di iodo tyrosine).
- **Coupling:** Coupling of 2 DIT will lead to the formation of T_4 and 1 MIT with 1 DIT will results in T_3.

After the synthesis, the hormone with thyroglobulin gets stored in the colloid.

List of antithyroid drugs (Table 4.6)

Table 4.6 List of antithyroid drugs

1. Perchlorates and thiocyanates negatively charged. Compete with iodides
2. Thiouracil group of drugs inhibit peroxidase enzyme activity
3. Iodides in high (mg) dosage

At the time of release of the hormones into circulation, the acinar cells will engulf the thyroglobulin along with the hormones by endocytosis.

In the cells the hormone will be separated by proteolysis and released into the circulation and thyroglobulin will be retained for further use.

Most of the hormone in circulation is in the protein bound form along with thyroid binding globulin (TBG), albumin and thyroid binding prealbumin.

Actions of the hormone

1. Calorigenic action

- Increases the oxygen consumption in almost all the tissues of the body except adult brain, gonads, lymphoid tissue. Increased metabolic rate increases the heat production in the body. The unit to measure heat energy is calorie.
- In normal adult male the basal metabolic rate (BMR) is about 40 Kcal/sq m BSA/Hr ± 15%.
- In hyperthyroidism it can be as much as + 60 to 100 %.
- In hypothyroidism it can fall by - 40 to 60 %.
- Hence estimation of BMR forms one of the thyroid function tests.

2. Nervous system (Table. 4.7)

- For the growth of the nervous system in the first 3 years of the postnatal period the action of the thyroxine on brain is essential. The growth of the brain occurs only during this phase.

The growth of the brain includes

- Formation of the synapses
- Growth of axon and dendrites and arborisation of these processes
- Increase in the number of glial cells
- **Myelination of nerve fibers**

Table 4.7 List of CNS features in thyroxine deficiency in infancy

1. The brain remains small
2. Number and size of the nerve cells reduced.
3. Arborization of the dendrites - less profuse
4. Myelination - Defective
5. CSF - Protein content is increased Net effect in human child I.Q.is markedly decreased.

Because of these reasons the action of hormone on the brain is very crucial in the first one to two years of postnatal life. If there is deficiency of the hormone during this period it can lead to mental retardation, one of the symptoms of which is the delayed milestones during the growth of the infant.

3. **On growth and development**

   It affects the growth and development of other parts of body as well.

   - The general growth is influenced by the growth hormone of the anterior pituitary gland but thyroxin potentiates the action of the growth hormone and hence the summated effect of these hormones is very much for the linear growth of the body and the growth of other organs.

   - It also affects the growth of reproductive organs and lack of the hormone may lead to sterility, infantile sex organs in adult, menstrual problems.

4. **Metabolic actions**: Apart from its action on the oxygen consumption by the tissues, it also influences the metabolism of carbohydrate, fats and proteins.

   a. **Carbohydrate metabolism:** acts as a hyperglycemic agent.

      - Increases the blood glucose level by increasing gluconeogenesis and glycogenolysis in the liver.

      - It also enhances the peripheral utilization of glucose.

   b. **Protein metabolism:** Has both anabolic and catabolic effects. Excess of hormonal level in circulaltion, catabolism predominates and leads to loss of body weight and muscular weakness. In hypothyroidism the anabolism suffers and again leads

to muscular weakness.

   c. **Fat metabolism:** Increases lipolysis. Cholesterol synthesis and degradation are both affected by this hormone. The degradation is more dependent on thyroxin than synthesis and hence in hypothyroidism the serum cholesterol level is increased.

   d. **On mucopolysaccharides:** The excretion of substances like hyaluronic acid and chondroitin sulphate is affected by the action of this hormone. Hence in hypothyroidism they get deposited in the sub cutaneous region-giving rise to myxoedema

5. **On systems:** The hormone affects functioning of the different systems of the body. Some of the systems on which the actions are more pronounced are

   a. **CVS**

      - It increases both the heart rate and force of contraction.

      - It increases the number of beta receptors and affinity of the beta-receptors for catecholamines.

      - Hence the resting heart rate will be more in hyperthyroid subjects. The increase in cardiac output leads to increase of systolic blood pressure (systolic hypertension).

      - It also increases the blood flow to the skin in order to facilitate the heat loss from the body. It is essential as the hormone increases basal metabolic rate and hence increased heat production.

   b. **GIT:** Hormone is required for normal secretory aspects and movements of gastro intestinal tract. In hyperthyroidism the patients suffer from diarrhoea and in hypothyroidism it is constipation.

   c. **Nervous system**

      In adult it affects the velocity of impulse conduction in the nerve fibers. In hyposecretion state it results in increased reflex time and vice versa in hyperthyroidism.

Regulation of secretion of hormone is brought about by the negative feed back mechanism. There is involvement of hypothalamo pituitary – thyroid axis (Fig. 4.2).

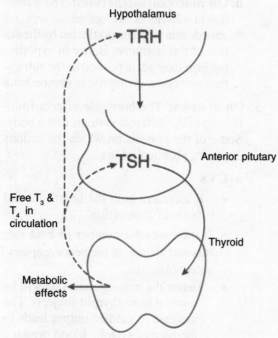

Fig 4.2 Regulation of secretion of hormone

Hypothalamus

TRH

TSH

Anterior pituitary

Free T₃ & T₄ in circulation

Thyroid

Metabolic effects

Increase in free form of hormone in circulation **acts on hypothalamus and anterior pituitary gland.** Acting on hypothalmus it decreases the secretion of thyrotropin releasing hormone (TRF) and acting on anterior pituitary decreases secretion of TSH.

Net effect will be decreased TSH from anterior pituitary gland. This decreases the secretion of thyroid hormones from the gland.

Alteration in the temperature can directly act on the hypothalamus to alter the secretion of the hormone.

Applied aspects

Physiologic basis for the features — see the actions.

Cretinism (Table 4.8)

Decreased thyroxin secretion in infancy and fetal life.

Table 4.8 Features of cretinism
• Are dwarfs
• Mentally retarded - low IQ
• Potbelly, Enlarged tongue
• Delayed mile stone
• Peculiar cry

Features are

• Stunted physical growth

• Mental retardation

• Pot belly

• Thick protruded tongue

• Sexual organ development suffers

• Developmental milestones get postponed

• Hoarse voice.

• Less active.

Myxoedema: Hypothyroidism in adults

Features are (Table 4.9)

• Decreased BMR

• Cold dry skin

• Hoarse voice

• Bradycardia & hypotension

• Cold dry skin with coarse and sparse hair

• Intolerance to cold

• Constipation

• Non-pitting edema due to the deposition of

osmotically active substances like hyaluronic acid and chondroitin sulphate in the subcutaneous tissue along with water.

Table 4.9 Features of myxedema

Myxoedema	- Hypothyrodism in adults
Problems may be with	- Thyroid gland
	pituitary gland
	Hypothalamus
SIGNS -	Low BMR
Hair	- coarse and sparse
Skin	- dry and yellow
Cold	- poorly tolerated
Voice	- hoarse
Mentation	- slow, sluggish

Thyrotoxycosis (Grave's disease, Exophthalmic goitre)

Hyperthyroidism in adult.

Features are (Table 4.10)

- Goitre (enlargement of thyroid gland)
- Increased BMR
- Weight loss due to degradation of proteins
- Extreme tachycardia
- Easy fatiguability
- Fine tremors
- Anxiety, nervousness

Table 4.10 Features of hyperthyroidism

- Nervousness
- Weight loss inspite of hyperphagia
- Heat intolerance
- Increased pulse pressure and heart rate
- Tremors - Fine
- BMR - ↑↑+60 to +100%
- Exophthalmos may be present

- Intolerance to heat
- Diarrhea.
- Warm wet skin

Thyroid function tests

- Estimation of BMR
- Estimation of serum cholesterol level
- Estimation of free T_3 & T_4, TSH
- Estimation of protein bound iodine (PBI)
- Uptake of iodine study by radio immuno assay.

CALCIUM METABOLISM

Calcium is one of the important inorganic ions present in all the tissues of the body. In a normal adult, about 1100 g of calcium is present and 99 % of this is in bones only.

- **Plasma calcium level is 9–11 mg%, of this 50% is in ionic form which is diffusible (4-5 mg%)**
- And the remaining 4-5 mg% will be in the bound form that is non diffusible (along with plasma proteins and as calcium salts).

The biologic action of calcium is because of the ionic form (Table 4.11).

Table 4.11 Calcium in the body

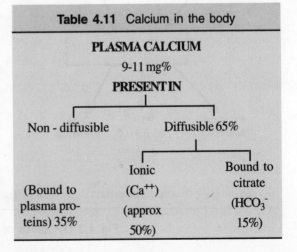

PLASMA CALCIUM

9-11 mg%

PRESENT IN

Non - diffusible (Bound to plasma proteins) 35%

Diffusible 65%

Ionic (Ca^{++}) (approx 50%)

Bound to citrate (HCO_3^- 15%)

Functions of ionic calcium (Table 4.12)

- Required to maintain the excitability of neurons and muscle by maintaing RMP.
- Required to maintain the excitability and contractility of cardiac muscle
- Necessary for neuromuscular transmission
- Acts as second messenger for certain hormonal actions

- Necessary for coagulation of blood
- Helps in the formation of bone and teeth

The daily intake of calcium is about 1000 mg. From the body there will be loss of about 900 mg/day along with the feces and about 100 mg/day along with the urine. During the growing periods of life, in pregnant and lactating female the requirement is more than 1000 mg/day. Calcium gets absorbed in the duodenum region and the acid medium facilitates the absorption (Fig. 4.3).

Bone physiology: Calcium and phosphate get deposited in the bone as hydroxyapatite crystals. Calcium in this state can't be removed from the bones. There will be continuous turnover of calcium present in the bone by osteoclastic activity, which releases calcium from bone and osteoblastic activity, which helps for deposition calcium salts on bones. Osteocytes pump bone calcium via the osteoblasts into the extracellular fluid.

Table 4.12 Functions of ionic calcium

1. Maintenance of resting membrane potential and hence excitability of nerve and muscle tissue
2. Release of ACh at N.M.J.
3. Excitation contraction coupling
4. Rhythmicity and contractility of cardiac muscle
5. Blood coagulation
6. Formation of bone and teeth
7. Release of certain hormones
8. Activation of certain enzyme (ATPase, lipase)
9. Formation of intercellular matrix (ground substance)

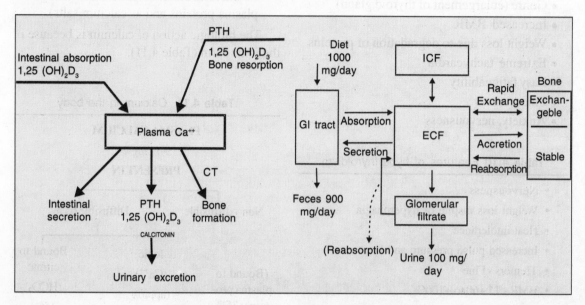

Fig 4.3 Dynamics of calcium in the body

Calcium metabolism is regulated in the body by 3 important hormones namely:

1. **Parathormone** secreted by the parathyroid gland, which is one of the essential endocrine glands. **The parathyroid glands are 4 in number present in the posterior aspect of thyroid gland at superior and inferior poles.**

2. **1–25 DHCC (dihydroxycholecalciferol) is the active form of vitamin D.**

3. **The para follicular cells of thyroid gland secrete calcitonin.**

Of the three, the first two are hypercalcaemic agents and the third is hypocalcaemic agent. Parathormone and calcitonin are peptide hormones and vitamin D is steroid in nature.

Actions of parathormone

On bone (Table 4.13)

Stimulates the activity of osteoclasts and inhibits the activity of osteoblasts. The release of cytokines will stimulate the osteoclastic activity. Due to this calcium and phosphate are liberated from the stable compartment of bone by a process known as resorption. The released calcium and phosphate will enter the circulation.

Table 4.13 Actions of PTH on bone
Directly acts
Bone resorption
-Mobilizes - Ca^{++}
PO_4-
By ↑Osteoclastic activity
↑The number of osteoclasts
Mechanism of action by increasing the production of cyclic AMP
(Through ↑Adenylate cyclase activity)

On kidney (Tables 4.14 and 4.15)

Exerts a number of actions to ensure that calcium level in circulation is increased but that of phosphate is decreased. This is essential in order to prevent the levels of these substance not to reach the solubility product. In case the level reaches the solubility product it will lead to deposition of calcium and phosphate on bones. The actions of parathormone on kidney are:

a. Increases the reabsorption of calcium from the distal convoluted tubule.

b. Increases the excretion of phosphate along with urine.

c. Stimulates the activity of the enzyme 1 alpha hydroxylase so that more amount of 1–25 DHCC is formed. The increased formation of vitamin D_3 facilitates absorption of calcium from the duodenum region of the intestine.

Table 4.14 Action of PTH on kidney
1. Increases reabsorption of Ca^{++} from DCT
2. Decreases the reabsorption of PO_4^- from PCT   Mechanism of action through increased formation of cyclic AMP
3. Increases the formation of 1,25 $(OH)_2CC$

Table 4.15 Indirect action of PTH on GIT
- Action is indirect through 1,25 (OH_2) DHCC
- Increases the absorption of Ca^{++}

Actions of calcitonin

It is the only hypocalcaemic agent.

Actions (Tables 4.16 & 4.17)

On bone

Enhances the deposition of calcium in the bone. This is brought about by increasing the osteoblastic activity and at the same time inhibiting the activity of the osteoclasts. So the calcium is removed from the circulation and deposited in the bones along with the phosphate.

On kidney

Acts on the distal convoluted and inhibits the reabsorption of calcium. So more calcium is excreted along with the urine.

Calcitonin is important in infants and children because the growth of bones has to occur in them in order to increase the mass and length of bone. In pregnant female the increase in calcitonin level in circulation prevents the removal of calcium from the bones of the mother for supply to the developing fetus.

1,25 DHCC (Schematic chart. 4.1)

This is another hypercalcaemic agent. It is the active form of vitamin D. It can get synthesized endogenously as well. When skin is exposed to the UV rays of sun light, 7-dehydrocholesterol present in the skin is converted to cholecalciferol. This is taken to the liver and converted to 25 - hydroxy cholecalciferol (25 HCC). 25 hydroxy chole calciferol is further taken to the kidney and converted to 1-25 di hydroxy chole calciferol (DHCC) by the action of 1- alpha hydroxylase (schematic chart 4.1).

Table 4.16 Actions of calcitonin
Calcitonin
lower Ca^{++} and $PO4^-$
Ca^{++} - is due to inhibition of bone resorption
- Inhibition of osteoclastic activity
- Increases Ca^{++} excretion in urine

Table 4.17 Physiologic importance of calcitonin
1. Hormone production is more in young -may play a role in skeletal development
2. May protect post-prandial hypercalcemia
3. Protect maternal bone during pregnancy and lactation and tendency towards bone loss during pregnancy

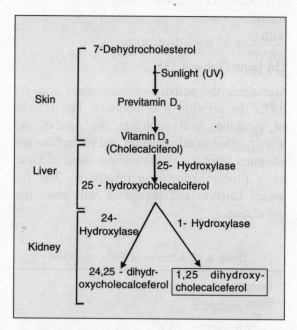

Schematic chart 4.1 Synthesis of vitamin D_3

Actions

On GIT

Acts on the duodenum and increases the absorption of calcium.

On bone

Osteocytes can pump calcium from the bone via the osteoblasts into the extracellular fluid compartment. The hormone also increases the osteocytes activity.

Regulation of secretion of parathormone and calcitonin (Fig. 4.4)

It is brought about by the concentration of calcium in circulation. More is calcium level in circulation more will be the secretion of calcitonin and when the calcium level falls, then there is increased secretion of parathormone.

Applied aspects

Hypoparathyroidism

Inadvertent removal of parathyroid glands along with thyroid gland during thyroidectomy causes hypoparathyroidism. **The signs and symptoms are due to decrease in calcium level.**

The symptoms are (Table 4.18)

- Increased neuromuscular excitability which causes tetany, manifested in the form of Chevostek's sign - tapping on facial nerve at angle of jaw leads to tetanic contractions of ipsilateral facial muscles.

- Trousseau's sign- on application of the blood pressure cuff and raising the pressure, patient may develop carpopedal spasm

- And in most severe case the patient may die of spasm of laryngeal muscles (laryngeal stridor and asphyxia).

Table 4.18 Features of hypocalcemic tetany

Characterised by increased neuro muscular excitability

1. Numbness, Tingling sesnsation of extremities - Paraesthesia
2. Stiffness in hands and feet
3. Cramps in extremities
4. Carpal spasm
   latent tetany
5. Convulsions in children
6. Laryngeal spasm (stridor)
7. Visceral manifestations

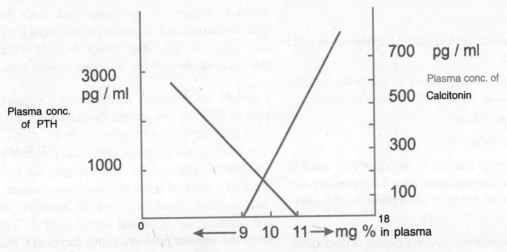

Fig. 4.4 Regulation of secretion of PTH and calcitonin

Tetany

Sustained painful contractions of the muscles. There are many factors which are responsible for onset of tetany. Tetany can also occur in diseases of kidney and in hyperventilation.

Equation indicating tendency to develop tetany

$$\text{Tendency to develop tetany} = \frac{[HCO_3^-][HPO_4^-]}{[H^+][Ca^{++}][Mg^+]}$$

There are two type of tetany:

a. Latent tetany in which there will not be any tetanic contractions at rest but seen when mild stimulus is applied.

b. Frank tetany where even in the absence of any stimuli there will be tetanic contractions.

Hyperparathyroidism

Tumors in bones cause release of calcium. As a result the bones become weak and are more susceptible for fracture. There will be depression of the activity of central nervous system.

Rickets

- Is caused due to vitamin D deficiency in child hood.
- Weight bearing bones in the body become weak and bowing of the bone may occur.
- Dental defects.
- Hypocalcaemia.

If there is vitamin D deficiency in adult it results in osteomalacia, which is normally due to decreased calcium absorption in the intestine.

Most common cause for rickets is inadequate exposure of skin to the sunlight.

ADRENAL GLANDS

The adrenals are made up of two parts. Outer zone known as adrenal cortex (an essential endocrine gland region) and the inner core region is adrenal medulla. The hormones secreted by adrenal cortex are collective known as cortico steroids whereas the medullary hormones are known as catecholamines. Apart from this difference, even during the embryonic life they get developed from entirely different regions and the medullary region is nothing but the modified ganglion of the sympathetic nervous system.

The adrenal cortex is divisible into 3 different layers; from outwards within will be

- Zona glomerulosa
- Zona fasciculata
- Zona reticularis.

All three layers secrete the hormones.

Zona glomerulosa secretes mineralocorticoids of which the most important is aldosterone.

Zona fasciculata and reticularis together secrete glucocorticoids of which the most important is cortisol & corticosterone. The layers also secrete sex steroids of which adrenal androgen is most important. Both the glucocorticoids and mineralocorticoids can exert the action of the other group as well when the concentration of the hormone is very high.

Cortisol is transported in circulation. A major part of it is in the protein bound form along with globulin (cortisol binding globulin –CBG). The level of this protein increases in pregnancy because of which in the initial stages, the free form of hormonal level in circulation decrease. This in turn stimulates more of secretion of the hormone by increased secretion of ACTH from the anterior pituitary gland. Level of CBG decreases in cirrhosis of liver and in nephrosis.

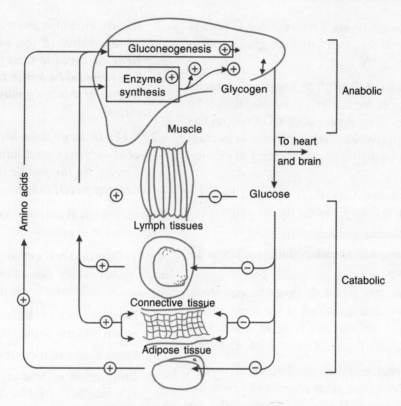

Fig 4.5 Metabolic actions of cortisol

Actions

1. Permissive action: Cortisol should be present in the target organs for the action of certain other hormones. For *example,* the catecholamines can exert the vasoconstrictor effect on vascular smooth muscle only in presence of cortisol. The vasoconstrictor effect is necessary to maintain peripheral resistance and hence blood pressure. Permissive action of cortisol is also required for certain actions of growth hormone and glucagon.

2. Metabolic actions (Fig. 4.5)

a. **Carbohydrate metabolism:** It is a hyper glycemic agent and increases blood glucose level

- By decreasing peripheral utilization of glu-

cose in almost all parts of body except heart and brain

- By increasing the gluconeogenesis and glycogenesis in liver.

- Excessive use of cortisol as therapeutic agent may lead to exhaustion of beta cells of pancreas and cause metasteroid diabetes.

b. **Protein metabolism:** In large doses it enhances the protein break down especially in the lymphoid tissue, muscles, bones.

- Leading to decreased immunity
- Muscular weakness
- Weight loss
- Susceptibility of the bones for fracture.

- The amino acids released due to protein break down are used for gluconeogenesis in the liver.

c. **Fat metabolism:** The hormone generally increases the lipolysis in adipose tissue. So brings about the break down of neutral fats and triglycerides. This will result in increase in free fatty acids and glycerol in circulation.

  - The free fatty acids are used both for energy supply to the tissues and
  - Gluconeogenesis in the liver.
  - There will be redistribution of fats in the body.
  - Fats are removed from the peripheral parts and deposited in the more central parts of body resulting in moon face, buffalo hump & pendulous abdomen.

d. **Mineral metabolism:** Excess of cortisol can also exert some amount of action like aldosterone. Hence it increases the sodium reabsorption in the distal convoluted tubule and in exchange for this potassium excretion in the urine increases. Reabsorpiton of sodium increases water retention, so blood volume and blood pressure get increased.

e. **Water metabolism:** Person with low levels of cortisol has defective water regulation in the body may be because the increase in the plasma anti diuretic hormone level and decreased glomerular filtration rate. Both of these con-tribute for delayed water excretion. The retention of water by the body can lead to water intoxication.

On organs

1. **CNS:** Increases the activity of the neurons in central nervous system and hence the patient may have euphoria. It will also increase the irritation of neurons and because which administration of this *as drug to any patient susceptible to/suffering from epilepsy should be borne in mind. Administration of this drug may worsen the condition.*

2. **GIT:** *In large dose increase the gastric acid secretion and damages the mucus barrier. So the people are more prone to develop peptic ulcer.*

Pharmacological actions occur only when the levels are far in excess.

Anti-inflammatory action: In some people acute inflammation can cause more damage to the tissues. Inflammation is due to increased

a. Blood flow due to increased metabolic rate of the bacteria at the site of infections

b. Permeability of the capillaries

c. Emigration of leucocytes to the site of infection from the blood vessels

d. Lysozyme release from the cells leading to proteolysis.

Cortisol counters the aforesaid effects by decreasing

a. Metabolic rate of bacteria

b. Capillary permeability

c. Emigration of leucocytes and stabilizing the lysozymes.

Cortisol should never be administered alone in bacterial infection as anti-inflammatory agent. It should always be combined with antibiotics to take care of the bacteria otherwise it can lead to spread of the bacteria, without the overt reaction of the body due to infection. This can lead to severe problems.

Anti-allergic activity

Especially in organ or tissue transplantation sometimes the recipient's body resists or rejects the new organ/tissue. Cortisol can be used to decrease the immuno suppression reactions. This helps to prevent rejection of the transplanted tissues.

Suppresses immune responses by

- Decreasing the eosinophil, lymphocyte and basophil count.
- Decreasing the eosinophil count by sequestration of the cells in liver and spleen.
- Decreasing the lymphocyte percentage by catabolism of proteins in lymphoid tissue. Hence it will decrease the concentration of circulating antibodies in course of time.

Regulation of secretion (Fig. 4.6)

By the negative feed back mechanism and there is involvement of hypothalamo-pituitary-adrenal axis. Increase free form of hormone in circulation acts on hypothalmus and anterior pituitary gland. From the hypothalamus secretion of corticotropin releasing factor (CRF) decreases, so it leads to decreased secretion of ACTH. Cortisol also acts directly on the anterior pituitary gland and inhibits secretion of ACTH. Decreased ACTH leads to less of cortisol secretion from the adrenal gland. Apart from this, stress and circadian rhythm directly act on hypothalamus to alter the secretions.

Cortisol as a drug when used one has to be careful at the time of discontinuation of the drug. Unlike any other drug, which can be stopped all of a sudden, this can't be done with cortisol. When exogenous cortisol is administered, the increased level of free form of cortisol in circulation

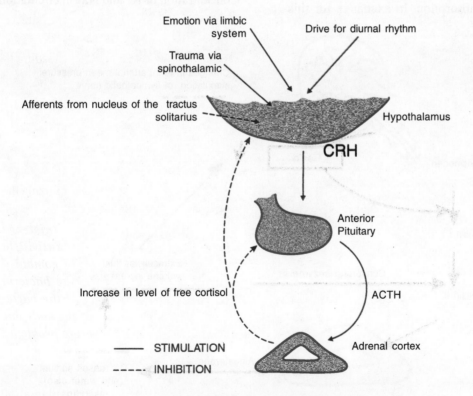

Fig 4.6 Regulation of secretion of cortisol

constantly inhibits the hypothalamus. This brings about the depression of the hypothalamo pituitary adrenal axis function. If cortisol is withdrawn suddenly the axis can't get revived immediately and patient may develop a crisis. If cortisol is withdrawn slowly and steadily (tapering dose) more time is provided for the regaining of the activity of the hypothalamo pituitary adrenal axis and the restoration of the endogenous secretion of cortisol can start once again.

Aldosterone

As stated already the most important mineralocorticoid is aldosterone, which is secreted by the zona glomerulosa.

Actions

On the kidney

Acts on the distal convoluted tubule and increases the sodium reabsorption. In exchange for this there will be increased secretion of either the potassium or hydrogen ion. Sodium reabsorption will be coupled with chloride and water reabsorption as well. This will increase the extra cellular fluid volume and hence blood volume.

On the epithelial cells of the kidney when aldosterone acts, it facilitates the Na^+—K^+ pump activity at the basolateral surface and increases the activity of the carrier proteins at the luminal surface.

On secretions

Decrease the amount of sodium lost along with the secretions like saliva and sweat in the body. So sodium loss from the body is minimized.

Regulation of secretion (Fig.4.7)

   a. Concentration of K^+ and Na^+ in circulation

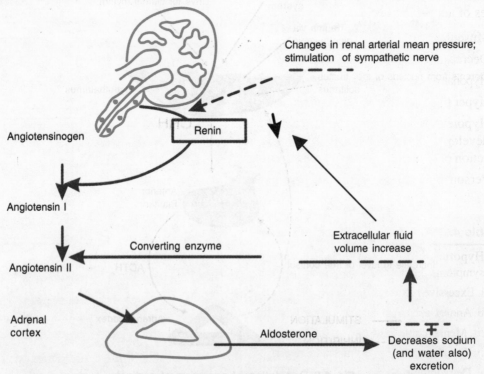

Fig 4.7 Regulation of secretion of aldosterone by renin angiotensin system

can act directly on the gland to alter the secretion. Of the two, the most potent is increase in the concentration of potassium. The normal plasma K$^+$ level is low (5 mEq/L water) when compared to Na$^+$ (150 mEq/L water). So small alteration in K$^+$ level will have a profound effect on the rate of secretion.

b. Angiotensin II: Which is formed due to activity of renin-angiotensin system can directly act on the adrenals and enhance the secretion of the hormone.

c. Some of the other factors which can increase the secretion of aldosterone, are anxiety, physical trauma and hemorrhage.

Applied aspects

Addison's disease (Table 4.19)

In this there is decreased secretion of all the hormones of adrenal cortex. The symptoms are:

- Muscular weakness.
- Decrease of blood pressure
- Hyponatremia, hyperkalemia and hypovolemia.
- Hyper pigmentation of skin and gums.
- Hypotension and person is susceptible to develop shock due the loss of permissive action of cortisol for catecholamine actions.
- Person is unable to withstand any stress, develops severe hypoglycemia when starved and may collapse.

Cushing's syndrome (Table 4.20)

Is due to hypersecretion of cortisol. Some of the important features are:

- Moon face and buffalo hump due to the centripetal distribution of fats.
- Muscle development is poor in hands and legs.
- Poor wound healing and more prone to infections.
- Negative nitrogen balance and muscle wasting.
- Pendulous abdomen and abdominal striae.
- Bruisability and ecchymoses.
- Increased bone dissolution may lead to osteoporosis.

Table 4.20 Features of Cushing's syndrome

Cushing Syndrome - ↑ **cortisol secretion**
Redistributiom of fat - Moon face, Buffalo hump, Pendulous abdomen
• Thin extremities - Protein catabolism
• Poor wound healing
• Muscular weakness
• Personality changes
• Hyperglycemic
• Hypertension

Conn's syndrome (Table 4.21)

Is due to primary hyperaldosteronism. There will be hyperplasia in the zona glomerulosa of adrenal cortex. Some of the important features are:

- Hypernatremia, hypokalemia and hypertension.

Table 4.19 Features of Addison's disease

I. Hypofunction-Addison's disease signs and symptoms due to ↓Aldosterone and ↓cortisol
i. Excessive pigmentation (due to ACTH)
ii. Anorexia, Nausea, Diarrhoea and Vomiting
iii. Mental confusion
iv. Decreased ability to withstand stress
v. Dehydration, Hypotension, Loss of weight

- Severe alkalosis.
- Osmotic diuresis due to increased excretion of sodium (because of sodium escape phenomenon) in the urine, the volume of urine excreted increases.
- Imbalance in the electrolyte concentration decreases the excitability of the tissue and hence leads to muscular weakness.
- Tendency to develop tetany due to alkalosis.
- Paradoxical aciduria due to increased excretion of hydrogen ion in exchange for sodium ion reabsorbed, though the pH of blood is more alkaline.

Table 4.21 Features of Conn's syndrome

CONN'S SYNDROME ↑ALDOSTERONE SECRETION
Hypertension (Hypernatremia)
Hypokalemia
Polyuria, Polydypsia
Alkalosis
Muscular weakness

Adrenal medulla

Secretes the hormones of emergency. The secretion is stimulated in conditions like fight, flight or fright. For the synthesis of the hormone the amino acid required is phenylalanine. Catecholamine group includes the hormones adrenaline, noradrenaline and dopamine. In human beings about 80% of the hormone secreted from this region is adrenaline.

Most the hormone will be degraded in the target organs and the end products of the metabolites are excreted along with the urine in the form of vanilyl mandelic acid and as conjugates.

The receptors through which the hormone acts are termed as adrenergic receptors. The types of receptors are alpha and beta. They are further divided into alpha 1 and alpha 2 and beta 1 and beta 2. The action of the hormone on the target organ depends on the type of receptor through which the action is mediated.

Actions (Table 4.22)

- **On vascular smooth muscle** (Fig 4.8):

  In presence of cortisol it is able to act on the smooth muscle of blood vessels especially in the arteriolar regions. Due to this some amount of vasoconstriction is maintained all the time and hence peripheral resistance. Peripheral resistance is the factor that is responsible for the diastolic blood pressure. Noradrenaline is a powerful vasoconstrictor.

- **On heart:** Is able to increase both the heart rate and force of contraction. Hence it increases cardiac output and systolic blood

Table 4.22 Comparative actions of adrenaline and noradrenaline

Norepinephrine	Parameters	Epinephrine
Decreased (due to reflex bradycardia)	Cardiac output	Increased
Increased	Periheral resistance	Decreased
++++	Mean arterial pressure elevation	+
++++	Free fatty acid release	+
++++	Stimulation of CNS	+++
+++	Increased heat production	++++
+	Increased blood sugar	++++
+	Dilation of bronchioles	++++

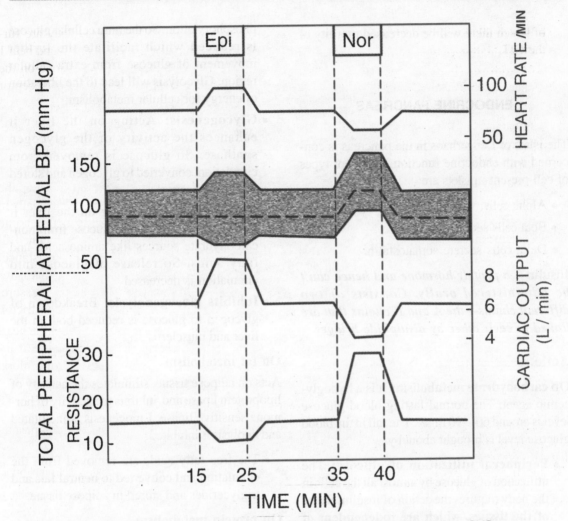

Fig 4.8 Comparative actions of adrenaline and noradrenaline on CVS

pressure in general.

- **On brain :** Increases the activity of the neurons of central nervous system and person becomes more alert.

- **On bronchial smooth muscle:** Brings about the broncho dilation and relieves a person suffering from bronchial asthma.

- **On iris:** Acts on the dilator pupillae muscle and hence there will be dilation of the pupil.

- **Metabolic effects:** Acts as hyperglycemic agent and increase blood glucose level by stimulating the glycogenolysis in the liver and muscle.

- It also increases the lipolysis and increases the free fatty acid release and also the metabolic rate of the tissue. Since it enhances the rate of metabolism it is termed as a calorigenic agent.

- **GIT:** Stimulates the activity of the sphincters and relaxes the smooth muscle because of which there will be decreased motility of the GIT.

ENDOCRINE PANCREAS

The islets of Langerhans in the pancreas is concerned with endocrine function. Different types of cell present in islets are

- Alpha cells, which secrete glucagon
- Beta cells secrete insulin
- Delta cells secrete somatostatin.

Insulin *is a peptide hormone and hence can't be administered orally. Consists of two different chains—the A and B chains that are linked to each other by disulphide bridges.*

Actions

On carbohydrate metabolism: It is a hypoglycemic agent. The normal fasting blood glucose level is around 60—90 mg%. The fall in the blood glucose level is brought about by

- **Peripheral utilization of glucose:** The utilization of glucose by almost all the cells in the body requires the action of insulin. **Some of the tissues, which are independent of insulin action for their glucose metabolism are**
- Whole of brain except satiety center in hypothalamus
- RBCs
- Intestinal mucosa
- Renal tubules.

  Insulin facilitates the movement of glucose from extra cellular compartment to intra cellular compartment and also increases the process of glycolysis in the cells. There will be increased activity of glucokinase and

phosphorylation. So the intra cellular glucose is reduced which facilitate the further movement of glucose from extra cellular region. Glycolysis will lead to the liberation of energy for cellular metabolism.

- **Glycogenesis:** Acting on the liver it enhances the activity of the glycogen synthase. So glucose is removed from circulation, converted to glycogen and stored in liver and muscles.
- **Gluconeogenesis:** Acting on the liver it inhibits the formation of glucose from non-carbohydrate sources like amino acids and fatty acids. So release of glucose into circulation is decreased.
- **Inhibits glycogenolysis:** Breakdown of glycogen to glucose is reduced both in the liver and muscle.

On fat metabolism

Acts on adipose tissue. stimulates the activity of lipoprotein lipase and inhibits the activity of hormone sensitive lipase. Lipogenesis is facilitated and lipolysis is inhibited.

- The free fatty acids are removed from the circulation and converted to neutral fats and triglycerides and stored in adipose tissue.

On protein metabolism

It is not only anabolic but also anti catabolic. So enhances the protein synthesis and decreases the protein degradation.

- The amino acids are removed from circulation and transferred into intra cellular fluid region.
- Inside the cells the amino acids are used for synthesis of proteins.
- Because of this the nitrogen content of the body increases.
- The increased protein synthesis facilitates the growth of the body in general and also helps for proper immune responses in the body by

maintaining the antibody production.

On potassium: It also increases the movement of potassium from outside the cell into inside the cell. Because of this when patients are on large doses of insulin therapy, there are chances developing hypokalemia. Giving extra amount of potassium can prevent development hypokalemia.

Regulation of secretion

It is always regulated by the substrate concentration in circulation. The level of glucose in the plasma directly acts on the beta cells and alters the secretion of insulin.

An increase of blood glucose level shall stimulate the secretion of insulin.

In addition to this some of the other factors which can also affect the secretion of insulin are, increase in the

- **Amino acids in circulation**
- **Free fatty acids in circulation and**
- **Stimulation of parasympathetic nerve.**
- **On the other hand somatostatin secreted by the delta cells inhibit the secretion of insulin.**

Diabetes mellitus (Table 4.23)

Deficiency of insulin generally causes diabetes mellitus. In diabetes either there can be absolute deficiency of insulin or the responsiveness of tissue is decreased for the action of insulin.

Some of the features of diabetes are:

a. **Hyperglycemia:** Increase of fasting blood glucose level.

b. **Glycosuria:** When blood glucose level exceeds the renal threshold of 180 mg% glucose starts getting excreted in the urine (Glycosuria).

c. **Polyuria:** Since glucose is an osmotically active substance, excretion of glucose will be coupled with excretion more volume of water (Polyuria).

d. **Polydypsia:** As body is losing more water, body water content decreases. This stimulates the thirst center and person drinks more water.

e. **Polyphagia:** The whole of central nervous system does not require insulin for glucose utilization except for satiety center in hypothalamus. The satiety center continuously inhibits the activity of hunger center as long as blood glucose level and insulin actions are normal. In diabetes, the glucose entry to satiety center decreases. This leads to no inhibition of the hunger

---

Table 4.23 Indicating features of diabetes mellitus

Signs and Symptoms of Diabetes Mellitus

1. Hyperglycemia - high blood glucose level. Normal fasting blood glucose 60-90 mg%

2. Followed by glycosuria

   Excretion of glucose in urine

   Renal threshold for glucose is 180 mg%

   Tubular maximum for glucose (Tm)

   -375 mg/min

Glycosuria-presence of glucose in urine

Polyuria, Polydypsia, Polyphagia

Weight loss inspite of Polyphagia

III. Early fatigue, weakness, loss of body weight, Poor growth

IV. Delayed wound healing, Repeated infection (carbuncles, furuncles)

   Due to negative nitrogen balance

V. Loss of fat sparing action of insulin results in

- More of lipolysis, decreased lipogenesis

   Therefore formation of ketone bodies (acetone, acetoacetic acid, beta hydroxybutyric acid)

center by the satiety center. The unopposed action of the hunger center results in polyphagia.

f. **Poor wound healing and resistance to infection decreases** because of negative nitrogen balance. Protein catabolism exceeds the protein anabolism. The antibody concentration in circulation also decreases. The increased protein catabolism leads to loss of weight and muscular weakness.

g. **Ketone body formation:** When glucose is unable to be utilized for the energy supply, free fatty acids released from the adipose tissue are metabolized to supply energy. So the ketone body production increases and person may suffer from keto acidosis.

Insulin excess will lead to hypoglycemia.

Some of the symptoms are

- Palpitation
- Sweating
- Nervousness due to increased autonomic nerve discharge, confusion,
- Lethargy, convulsions, coma and death.

Glucagon

The alpha cells of islets of Langerhans secrete glucagon hormone. Unlike insulin it is a hyperglycemic hormone. This hormone is also a peptide hormone.

Actions

Carbohydrate metabolism

Increases blood glucose level. This is brought about by its action on liver and muscle.

Both in liver and muscle it stimulates glycogenolysis and glucose is released into circulation due to glycogen break down. In the liver it will also stimulate gluconeogenesis and hence glucose is synthesized from non-carbohydrate sources.

Fat metabolism

Stimulate the activity of hormone sensitive lipase.

Increases lipolysis by acting on adipose tissue. Free fatty acids are released into circulation. Increased utilization of fatty acids to supply energy leads to more of ketone body formation.

On heart

The action occurs only when in large doses. Has got inotropic effect. So increases the force of contraction of myocardium.

Regulation of secretion (Table. 4.24)

Like insulin, the level of glucose in circulation also influences glucagon secretion. An increase of blood glucose level inhibits the secretion of glucagon. Other factors which can affect the secretions are

- **Somatostatin**
- **Sympathetic stimulation.**

Table 4.24 Factors affecting glucagon secretion

Stimulators	Inhibitors
Amino acids (particularly the glucogenic amino acids alamine, serine, glycine, cysteine and threonine)	Glucose
	Somatostatin
	Secretin
CCK, Gastrin	FFA
Cortisol	Insulin

Coma occurs both in hyperglycemic and in hypoglycemic state. The best way to deal with the comatose patient when you do not know the glycemic state is, administer glucose. If coma is because of hypoglycemia, the patient regains consciousness when blood glucose level increases. If the coma is because of hyperglycemia, the comatose state continues and administration of glucose will not cause any harm. Whether coma is because of hyper/hypoglycemic state can be ascertained by this without any further waste of time.

ANTERIOR PITUITARY (ADENOHYPOPHYSIS)

Situated in the sella turcica of the sphenoid bone. It is made up two important parts namely the anterior and posterior pituitary gland. Anterior pituitary is also known as adenohypophysis and posterior pituitary is known as neurohypophysis.

Anterior pituitary gland: Contains cells which are known as chromophobes and chromophils. The hormones secreting cells are chromophils (Table 4.25). The chromophils are further divided into acidophils and basophils. **The hormones secreted by the anterior pituitary are**

a. GH (growth hormone) or somatotropin

b. ACTH (for adrenal cortex) Adreno cortico tropic hormone

c. TSH (for thyroid) Thyroid stimulating hormone

Table 4.25 Cell types and hormones secreted

Cells - Somatotropes - GH
Lactotropes   - Prolactin
Thyrotropes   - TSH
Gonadotropes   - FSH & LH
Corticotropes - ACTH, endorphin and
                 βLPH   (Lipotropins)

d. FSH, LH (ICSH) (for gonads and these hormones together are known as gonado- tropic hormones): Follicular stimulating hormone and leutinizing hormone

e. Prolactin.

Connection of anterior pituitary gland with the hypothalamus (Schematic chart 4.2) is through hypothalamohypophyseal portal system. It is a vascular connection. From the

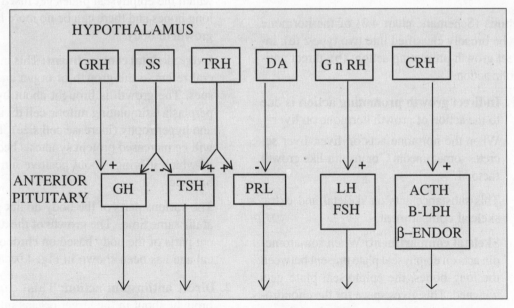

Regulation of anterior pituitary cell function by hypothalamic neurohormones. DA- dopamine, GH- growth hormone, SS - somatostatin, LPH-lipotropins, ENDOR- endorphins.

Schematic chart 4.2 Hypothalamic influence on anterior pituitary secretions

median eminence region of the hypothalamus there will be secretion of certain substances known as releasing or release inhibiting factor or hormone. When these factors/hormones reach the anterior pituitary through the portal circulation they alter the secretion from the anterior pituitary gland.

For example, when GRF/GRH is secreted from the hypothalamus, it stimulates growth hormone secretion from the anterior pituitary gland and if growth hormone secretion has to be inhibited, then hypothalamus secretes somatostatin. Because of this the hypothalamus-pituitary and the concerned gland axis forms one of the important mechanisms for the regulation of secretion of hormone.

Growth hormone

Is a peptide hormone secreted by the acidophils. As the name indicates its action is on the growth of the body.

Actions (Schematic chart 4.3) of the hormone can be broadly classified into two types: (a). indirect growth promoting action; (b). direct anti-insulin action.

1. **Indirect growth promoting action** is due to the action of growth hormone on liver

   When the hormone acts on liver, liver secretes somatomedin C or insulin-like growth factor I.

   This substance acts on skeletal and extra, skeletal compartment.

   Skeletal compartment: When somatomedin acts on epiphyseal plate present between the long bones, the epiphyseal plate gets widened. This gives space for the chondrogenesis of the long bones. The long bones grow linearly. Hence the height of the person increases. The long bones can grow only upto the age of about 18-20 years beyond

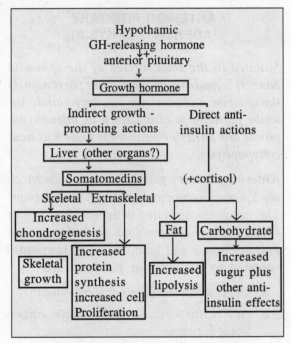

Schematic chart. 4.3 Actions of GH

which the epiphyseal plates get fused with long bones and there can be no more linear growth of body.

Extra skeletal compartment: This in general refers to the growth of organ and tissues. The growth is brought about by hyperplasia (stimulating mitotic cell division) and hypertrophy (increase cell size). There will be increased protein synthesis because of which it brings about positive nitrogen balance.

The various parts of the body do not grow at the same time. The growth of the different parts of the body based on chronological age has been shown in Fig. 4.9.

2. **Direct antiinsulin action:** This can be brought about in the target organs in presence of cortisol (permissive action of cortisol is required).

On carbohydrate metabolism: It is a hy-

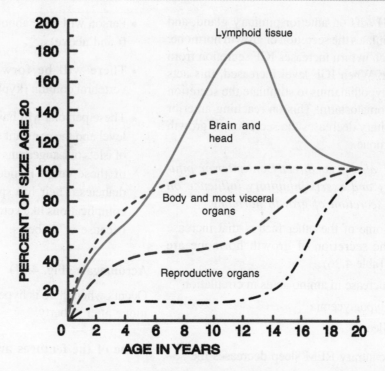

Fig 4.9 Growth of different parts of body

perglycemic agent. Increases the blood glucose level by

a. Decreasing the peripheral utilization of glucose.

b. Increased gluconeogenesis in liver.

Fat metabolism Acts on the adipose tissue. Neutral fats and triglycerides are broken down to release the free fatty acids. They are utilized for energy supply to the tissues. This can lead to increased production of keto acids.

Growth hormone also promotes the retention of sodium, potassium, calcium and phosphate since these substances are required for the growth of the body.

Regulation of secretion (Fig. 4.10) is mainly by the feedback control by the free form of the hormone level in circulation.

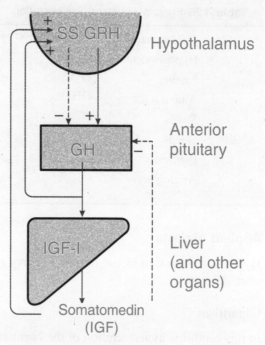

Fig 4.10 Regulation of secretion of GH

GRH acts on anterior pituitary gland. and stimulates the secretion of growth hormone, which in turn increases IGF secretion from liver. When IGF level increased, this acts on hypothalamus to stimulate the secretion of somatostatin. This on reaching anterior pituitary decreases the secretion of growth hormone.

IGF also acts directly on anterior pituitary and exerts inhibitory influence on the secretion of growth hormone.

Some of the other factors that increase the secretion of growth hormone are (Table 4.26)

- Increase in amino acids in circulation
- Hypoglycemia
- Sleep

On the contrary REM sleep decreases the secretion.

Table 4.26 Factors affecting GH secretion

Factors	↑GH secretion by	↓GH secretion by
	Hypoglycemia	Cortisol
	Fasting	FFA
	Amino acids	GH
	Stress	
	Sleep	
	Estrogens	
	Androgens	

Applied aspects

Hypersecretion: Can occur before puberty or after puberty.

Gigantism

In this condition hypersecretion of the hormone occurs right from childhood.

- Person will have abnormal height (around 8 ft and above).

- There will be forward bending of the vertebral column (kyphosis).

- These persons will have high blood glucose level and the constant stress on the beta cells of islets of Langerhans will lead to exhaustion of these cells. Hence they develop early diabetes. Their life span is limited due the complications like ketoacidosis they develop because of diabetes.

Acromegaly (Fig. 4.11)

Occurs when there is hyper secretion of the hormone after puberty.

Some of the features are

- Enlargement of acral parts hand and feet, as the long bones can't grow after puberty due to ossification.

- Prognatism: Enlarged mandible. Protrusion of the mandible occurs.

- Bitemporal hemianopia: Enlarged pituitary gland compresses the optic chaisma. So the person suffers from bi temporal hemianopia (loss of temporal half of field of vision in both the eyes).

- Osteoarthritic changes in the vertebral column.

- Hirsutism: Increased growth of hairs on the trunk.

- Gynaecomastia and lactation: There can be enlargement of breasts in male and at times milk secretion can also occur. This is because growth hormone to a certain extent can also act like prolactin.

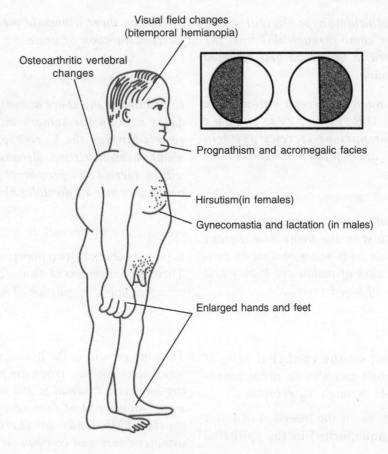

Visual field changes
(bitemporal hemianopia)

Osteoarthritic vertebral
changes

Prognathism and acromegalic facies

Hirsutism(in females)

Gynecomastia and lactation (in males)

Enlarged hands and feet

Fig. 4.11 Features of acromegaly

Dwarfism: Decreased growth hormone secretion in childhood.
Some of the features are:

- **Short stature** due to the failure of growth of the long bones.

- **No mental retardation:** Unlike thryroxine, which is essential for the growth of central nervous system in the first few years of postnatal life, growth hormone does not have influence on developement of brain. Milestones of development remain normal.

- **Sexual growth:** Occurs normally in these individuals and hence generally they have the ability to reproduce.

POSTERIOR PITUITARY OR NEUROHYPOPHYSIS

The hormones of posterior pituitary gland get synthesized in the neurons of the hypothalamus. The two different groups of neurons in the hypothalamus, which synthesize these hormones, are supra optic and para ventricular nuclei (they are also known as magno cellular neurons in general).

The hormones get transported to the posterior pituitary gland from the hypothalamus through the axoplasmic flow. Supraoptic and paraventricular nuclei of the hypothalamus are connected to the posterior pituitary gland through hypothalamohypophyseal tract. When impulses come through this tract the hormones stored in the gland gets released into the circulation.

Supraoptic nucleus secretes anti-diuretic hormone(ADH/vasopressin)and paraventricular nucleus secretes oxytocin hormone. Both are peptide hormones.

Actions of Anti diuretic hormone

As the name indicates it decreases the volume of water lost in the urine and thereby helps to maintain body water content by conservation. The sites of action are kidney and smooth muscle of blood vessels:

Water reabsorption

- **It acts most on the epithelial cells of collecting duct and also on distal convoluted tubule through V_2 receptors.**

- **This brings about the insertion of water channels (aquaporins) in the epithelial cells.**

- **Through these channels water gets reabsorbed.**

- **Most the water reabsorbed in these regions of the kidney is under the influence of this hormone.**

Urea movement

Facilitates the rate of urea getting recycled from the collecting duct through the interstitial region of renal medulla back into the fluid in the ascending limb of loop of Henle.

Rate of blood flow through the vasa recta

It reduces the rate of blood flow through the vasa recta and helps for better functioning of the counter-current system.

All the three aforesaid mechanisms help for concentration of urine.

Vascular smooth muscle

In addition to the above actions, ADH in large doses acts on the smooth muscle of blood vessels through the V_1 receptors and brings about vasoconstriction. Because of this there will be increase in peripheral resistance and hence increase of diastolic blood pressure.

Regulation of secretion

Is brought about by two important mechanisms. There is involvement of osmoreceptors and volume receptors in regulation of secretion.

Osmoreceptors

They are present in the hypothalamus near the supra optic nucleus. *When the plasma osmolality increases (normal is 300 mosm/L water), water moves out of osmoreceptors by exosmosis. This leads to shrinkage of the osmoreceptors and consequent stimulation of them. This in turn stimulates the supra optic nucleus. From the supra optic nucleus more impulses are sent to posterior pituitary through the hypothalamo hypophyseal tract. More anti diuretic hormone will be released into the circulation. This helps for retention of more water through the kidneys and normalizes the osmolality of the plasma.*

Volume receptors

Volume receptors are present in the walls of the great veins and on the right side heart. They are also known as low-pressure receptors. Increase in blood volume stimulates these receptors. Afferent impulses from the receptors reach the hypothalamus and inhibit the activity of supraoptic nucleus. So less anti-diuretic hormone is released from the poste-

rior pituitary gland into circulation. This decreases the volume of water reabsorbed from the renal tubules. Increased urine output will restore the blood volume.*

Some of the other factors that can alter secretion of the hormone are

- Alcohol
- Pain
- Surgery
- Trauma.

Applied aspect

Diabetes insipidus: **Occurs due to deficiency of anti-diuretic hormone secretion.**

Some of the features are

- **Polyuria:** *Increased volume of urine excretion due to loss of concentrating ability in kidney.*
- **Polydypsia:** *Increased thirst center activity due to decrease in body water content. Person drinks more water.*
- **Urine will not have glucose and blood glucose level will be normal.**
- **The specific gravity of the urine will be less due to excretion of more dilute urine most of the times.**

Oxytocin

This hormone is secreted by the para ventricular nucleus of hypothalamus.

Actions

On the breasts

Acts on the myoepithelial cells of the breasts. This causes the ejection of milk from the alveolar ducts of the breasts.

On myometrium

Acts on the myometrium of the uterus and causes severe contraction of the myometrium. This leads to the parturition or delivery of the fetus due to an increase in the intra uterine pressure.

In the non pregnant woman oxytocin is believed to bring about minute myometrial contractions which facilitates movement of sperm along the uterus to reach fallopian tubes.

In males, it is believed to bring about contraction of smooth muscles in vas deferens.

Regulation of secretion

Is brought about by a neuro endocrine reflex. In this reflex, part of the reflex pathway is neural and part is hormonal (Flow chart 4.1). Milk ejection and parturition reflexes are classical examples of neuro endocrine reflex.

Suckling of the breasts brings about the stimulation of the touch receptors present on the nipple and areola. Afferent impulses are carried to the hypothalamus through the ascending tracts of spinal cord and stimulate the para ventricular nucleus. Impulses coming along the hypothalamo hypophyseal tract bring about the release of the hormone from the post pituitary gland into the circulation. The hormone on reaching breasts brings about milk ejection by acting on the myoepithelial cells.

When head of the fetus presses on the cervix, the stretch receptors present in the cervix get stimulated and the afferent impulses go through the ascending tracts of spinal cord to reach hypothalamus. This brings about the stimulation of the paraventricular nucleus in the hypothalamus. More impulses go along the hypothalamohypophyseal tract to the posterior pituitary gland. This leads to the release of the hormone into circulation. The hormone acts on the myometrium present in the uterus to bring about contractions of the uterus resulting in parturition (delivery of fetus).

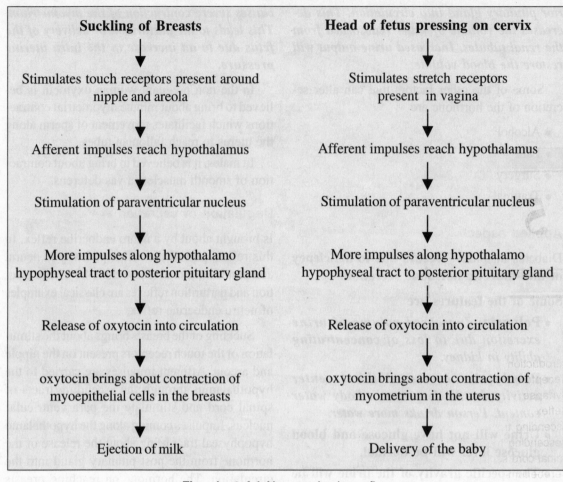

Suckling of Breasts	**Head of fetus pressing on cervix**
↓	↓
Stimulates touch receptors present around nipple and areola	Stimulates stretch receptors present in vagina
↓	↓
Afferent impulses reach hypothalamus	Afferent impulses reach hypothalamus
↓	↓
Stimulation of paraventricular nucleus	Stimulation of paraventricular nucleus
↓	↓
More impulses along hypothalamo hypophyseal tract to posterior pituitary gland	More impulses along hypothalamo hypophyseal tract to posterior pituitary gland
↓	↓
Release of oxytocin into circulation	Release of oxytocin into circulation
↓	↓
oxytocin brings about contraction of myoepithelial cells in the breasts	oxytocin brings about contraction of myometrium in the uterus
↓	↓
Ejection of milk	Delivery of the baby

Flowchart 4.1 Neuroendocrine reflex

Central Nervous System (CNS)

- Introduction
- Receptors
- Synapse
- Reflex
- Ascending tracts
- Descending tracts
- Spinal cord sectioning
- Cerebellum
- Basal ganglia
- Thalamus
- Vestibular appratus
- Hypothalamus
- Limbic system
- Cerebrospinal fluid
- Reticular formation
- Electroencephalo-gram
- Learning and memory
- Cerebral cortex
- Autonomic nervous system

INTRODUCTION AND BROAD DIVISION OF NERVOUS SYSTEM

- The nervous system is broadly divisible into CNS (Central nervous system) and PNS (Peripheral nervous system).
- CNS refers to brain and spinal cord.
- PNS includes all the nerves present in different parts of body other than CNS.

These peripheral nerves, *which carry impulses from the various parts of body to central nervous system*, are termed *afferent or sensory*.

The peripheral nerves *that carry impulses from the central nervous system to all the other parts of body* are called *efferent or motor*.

RECEPTORS

The specialized nerve endings in the peripheral parts of afferent nervous system are known as receptors. These receptors act as biologic transducers and convert any form of energy into an electrical activity (impulse) in the afferent nerve fibre.

The nature of energy (stimulus) can be

- Chemical
- Mechanical
- Thermal.

The afferent impulses are carried from different parts of body to the central nervous system and keep informing the central nervous system about the happenings in the peripheral parts of body.

Classification of the receptors

Can be done based on different criteria. One of the ways in which it can be classified will be as follows:

Based on the type of stimulus for which they respond, they can be classified into

- **Mechanoreceptors:** *Respond for mechanical energy like touch, pressure, vibration.* These receptors are present in almost all parts of body.

In skin there are (Fig. 5.1)

- Merkel's disc
- Meissner's corpuscle (touch receptors)
- Pacinian corpuscle etc.

In the visceral regions we come across

- Barorceptors
- Volume receptors
- Auditory receptors.

- **Chemoreceptors respond for chemical energy.** They are

- Taste receptors
- Olfactory receptors.
- Carotid and aortic bodies
- Osmoreceptors.

- **Themoreceptors** *get stimulated by thermal energy.* Thermoreceptors of skin (peripheral) and hypothalamus (central) are the examples.

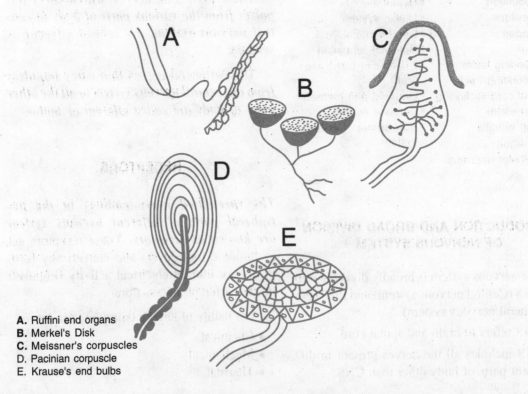

A. Ruffini end organs
B. Merkel's Disk
C. Meissner's corpuscles
D. Pacinian corpuscle
E. Krause's end bulbs

Fig. 5.1 Structure of different cutaneous receptors

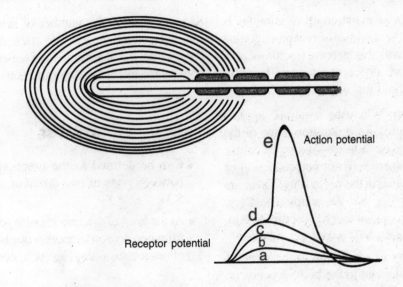

e — Action potential

d
c
b
a

Receptor potential

Fig. 5.2 Diagram of receptor potential in a pacinian corpuscle

- **Nociceptors** *get stimulated for the painful (noxious) stimulus.* The naked nerve endings present in almost all the parts of body act as nociceptors. They are absent in central nervous system.

- **Electromagnetic receptors** *present in the eye.* They respond for the light rays (electro magnetic waves). E.g. rods and cones (photoreceptors).

Properties

1. **Excitability**: Since receptors are specialized nerve endings they are also in the polarized state when not stimulated. On application of the stimulus, the change in the polarized state occurs, which leads to the development of receptor potential or generator potential. When the potential reaches a critical value there will be development of nerve action potential in the afferent fibre (Fig. 5.2).

2. **Adequate stimulus** is the just enough strength of stimulus to excite the receptor for the production of receptor potential.

When receptor potential reaches a certain value there will be development of action potential in the afferent fiber.

3. **Specificity:** Each group of receptor is specialized to respond for a particular type of stimulus very easily. However the same receptors can get stimulated for some other type of stimulus provided the strength of stimulus is very strong. E.g. photoreceptors are most sensitive to light but application of pressure on the eyeball can also stimulate them.

4. **Intensity discrimination:** The strength of stimulus applied can be assesed by the magnitude of response from the receptors in the form of increase in the amplitude of receptor potential. An increased amplitude of the receptor potential increases the number of action potentials in unit time, in the afferent nerve fibre as per Weber Fechner law (as per this law the frequency of action potential in the nerve fibre is directly proportional to log intensity of stimulus). Another way by which the intensity discrimination can be

made out is as the strength of stimulus is increased, the number of receptors getting stimulated will also increase (recruitment of receptors) as different receptors have diverse threshold for excitation.

5. **Adaptation:** When the stimulus applied acts for a prolonged duration some of the receptors may stop responding in course of time.So there will not be production of action potential in the nerve fibre. There are some receptors that get adapted fast e.g. olfactory receptors, touch receptors in skin. *Pain receptors will never get adapted*

- The property of adaptation of the receptor whether beneficial to the body depends on the type of receptor that has got adapted. Baroreceptor adaptation is detrimental to the body function as blood pressure cannot be restored to normal value during sustained hypertension as this group of receptor get adapted for higher pressure.

Sensory unit is the number of sensory receptors from which a particular afferent nerve fiber carries impulse. Recruitment of sensory units also help for the intensity discrimination.

SYNAPSE

- Can be defined as the functional junction between parts of two different neurons Fig. 5.3).

- At the level of synapse impulse get conducted from one neuron to another due to the release of neurotransmitter like ACh, nor adrenaline

- These types of synapses, which require the release of some chemical substance (neurotransmitter) during synaptic transmission are termed as chemical synapses. In the human body almost all the synapses are chemical type.

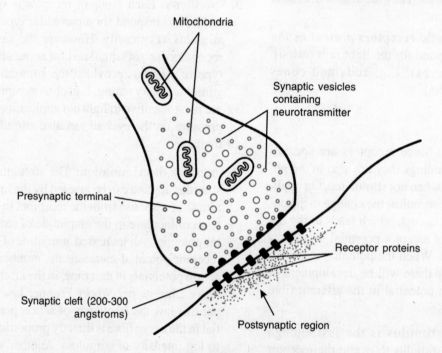

Fig. 5.3 Diagram of synapse

Labels in figure: Mitochondria; Synaptic vesicles containing neurotransmitter; Presynaptic terminal; Receptor proteins; Synaptic cleft (200-300 angstroms); Postsynaptic region

Parts involved in a synapse

Presynaptic region is mostly contributed by axon and postsynaptic region may be contributed by dendrite or soma (cell body) or axon.

Mechanism of synaptic transmission

a. Arrival of impulse

b. Presynaptic region getting depolarized

c. Release of neurotransmitter

d. Passage of neurotransmitter through synaptic cleft.

e. Binding of the neurotransmitter to receptors on postsynaptic region.

f. Change in the electrical activity of the postsynaptic region (EPSP or excitatory postsynaptic potential/IPSP or inhibitory postsynaptic potential also known as local potentials) leading to depolarisation/hyperpolarisation of the postsynaptic region.

g. Can be production or inhibition of the action potential generation. When EPSP reaches firing level, there will be generation of action potential in the postsynaptic region. EPSP is due to the influx of sodium ion and IPSP will be due to efflux of potassium or influx of chloride ion at the postsynaptic regions.

Properties of synapse (Table 5.1)

Table 5.1 Properties of synapses

1. Unidirectional conduction
2. Synaptic delay
3. Summation
4. Fatigue
5. Convergence and divergence
6. Inhibition/Excitation
7. Susceptible to H^+ changes, hypoxia and drugs

1. One-way conduction (unidirectional conduction): Since the neurotransmitter is present only in the presynaptic region the impulse can get conducted from pre to postsynaptic region only and not vice versa.

2. Synaptic delay is for the neurotransmitter to

- Get released from the synaptic vesicles
- Pass through the synaptic cleft
- Act on the postsynaptic region to elicit a response

some time is required. This is known as synaptic delay, which is normally about 0. 5 msec at each synapse.

3. Fatigability

When synapses get stimulated continuously, after some time due to the exhaustion of the neurotransmitter, the impulse fails to get conducted and causes fatigue. This is a temporary phenomenon, as the period of some mental rest given facilitates the resynthesis of neurotransmitter for further conduction of impulse.

4. Convergence and divergence

Impulses from the same presynaptic nerve fiber may end on the postsynaptic region of different neurons and this is called as **divergence**. When the nerve fibres of different presynaptic neurons end on a common postsynaptic neuron, this is known as **convergence.**

5. Summation

When a subthreshold stimulus is applied there will not be development of action potential in the postsynaptic region. But if many subthreshold stimuli are applied at the presynaptic region, the effects of these stimuli can get added up and lead to action potential development in the postsynaptic region. This is known as summation.

There are two types of summation namely spatial and temporal. In temporal summation the presynaptic neuron stimulated will be the same but many stimuli are applied in rapid suceession (timing of the stimuli will be different) but in spatial summation the presynaptic neurons stimulated will be different but the stimuli applied will be simultaneously (time of stimulation shall be same).

6. Excitation or inhibition

The impulse conduction across a synapse may either stimulate or inhibit the activity of the postsynaptic region. If there is stimulatory influence, then there will be production of action potential in the postsynaptic neuron and if it has an inhibitory influence, then there is no action potential generation in the postsynaptic region.

Examples of inhibition are

- Postsynaptic inhibition
- Presynaptic inhibition.
- Renshaw cell inhibition
- Reciprocal inhibition
- Lateral inhibition

Postsynaptic inhibition (Fig. 5.4)

Events during postsynaptic inhibition

a. Arrival of impulse at the presynaptic region.

b. Release neurotransmitter.

c. Stimulation of the internuncial neuron

d. Action potential production in the internuncial neuron

e. Release of neurotransmitter from internuncial neuron

f. Binding of neurotransmitter to receptors on postsynaptic region.

g. Influx of chloride ions into the postsynaptic region.

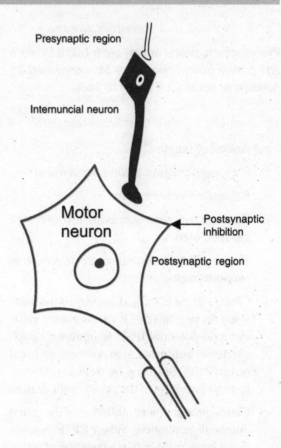

Fig. 5.4 Postsynaptic inhibition

h. Postsynaptic membrane becoming more negative (development of inhibitory postsynaptic potential or also known as IPSP).

i. Hyperpolarisation of postsynaptic region.

j. No action potential production in the postsynaptic region.

Glycine substance is a classical example of inhibitory neurotransmitter at postsynaptic region.

The mechanism of inhibition in all other types namely Renshaw cell, reciprocal and lateral, will be like what has been explained for the postsynaptic inhibition but the orientation of the neuron will be different.

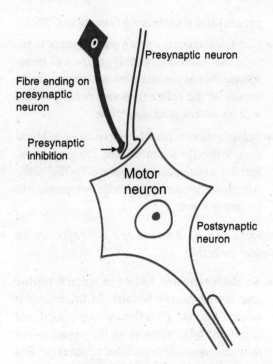

Fig. 5.5 Presynaptic inhibition

Presynaptic inhibition (Fig. 5.5)

In presynaptic inhibition the events are as follows:

a. The neuron ending on presynaptic terminal liberates neurotransmitter.

b. Because of this, the presynaptic terminal becomes more negative (either because of potassium efflux or chloride influx)

c. So there will be hyperpolarisation of the pre synpatic terminal.

d. Arrival of the action potential along the presynaptic terminal.

e. The depolarisation of the presynaptic terminal will not be to the extent it normally occurs in any other part of the neuron.

f. This leads to release of less than normal amount of neurotransmitter from the presynaptic terminals.

i. The neurotransmitter on binding to receptors on the postsynaptic region, brings about development of EPSP.

j. But the EPSP will be less and hence will not bring the postsynaptic region to threshold state of stimulation.

k. Hence there will not be production of action potential in the postsynaptic region.

REFLEX

Definition

Spontaneous/involuntary, stereotyped/repetitive, purpose serving response for afferent stimulation.

For any reflex action to be elicited the basic reflex arc should be intact.

The components of the basic reflex arc are (Fig. 5.6):

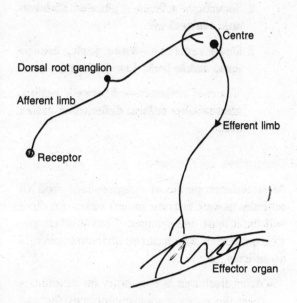

Fig. 5.6 Diagram of basic reflex arc

a. Receptor
b. Afferent limb
c. Center
d. Efferent limb
e. Effector organ.

Center can be present either in the brain or spinal cord. Damage to any part of the basic reflex arc results in loss of reflex activity in that part of the body.

Classification of reflexes *may be done based on different criteria.*

a. Unconditioned or conditioned *based on whether they are present by birth. Unconditoned is one which is present by birth*

b. Monosynaptic or polysynaptic *based on the number of synapses involved in the reflex activity.* Stretch reflex is the only monosynaptic reflex in the body.

c. **Clinical classification based on the location of the receptors which are involved in the reflex action:**

1. Superficial reflexes – **plantar, abdominal, corneal etc.**

2. Deep reflexes—**knee jerk, biceps jerk, ankle jerk, jaw jerk etc.**

3. Visceral reflexes— **Marey's reflex, micturition reflex, defecation reflex etc.**

Properties of reflexes

Most of the properties of synapses hold good for reflexes as well because in any reflex arc there will be at least one synapse. Certain other specific properties, which can be attributed specially to reflexes, are

- After discharge is even after the stimulus is over, the reflex response continues for prolonged duration. This is possible because of parallel and reverbrating circuits in CNS.

- Habituation occurs when the stimulus is benign (not harmful), initially there will be response, but as the stimulus continues, the intensity of the reflex response decreases and will be absent after sometime.

- Sensitization is just the opposite of habituation. When the stimulus is of dangerous one, for the subsequent exposure to the same stimulus, the intensity of reflex response will be much more.

Importance of knowledge of reflexes in clinical practice

- **To differentiate between upper motor and lower motor lesions.** In lower motor neuron lesions all reflexes (superficial and deep) are lost, whereas in the upper motor neuron lesions all superficial reflexes are lost except plantar reflex which is Babinski +ve and the deep reflexes get exaggerated. In cerebellar lesion the knee jerk (deep reflex) becomes pendular.

- **To assess the level of lesion in the CNS** For example, if reflexes are normal in upper half of body but altered or absent in lower half of body, it can be concluded that there is problem in the central nervous system of lower half of the spinal cord.

Plantar reflex (Fig. 5.7)

When sole of the foot is scratched firmly (may be with a key) in the lateral aspect from the heel towards the toes, the normal plantar response will be plantar flexion of all the toes. *In upper motor neuron lesion, there will be dorsiflexion of the great toe and fanning out (abduction) of the other toes. This response is known as Babinski +ve. In lower motor neuron or in afferent nerve lesions the plantar reflex shall be absent due to the damage in the basic reflex arc.*

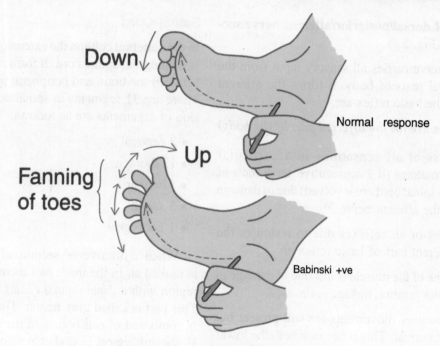

Down

Up

Fanning of toes

Normal response

Babinski +ve

Fig. 5.7 Plantar reflex normal and Babinski sign

Lower motor neuron is the anterior horn cell (AHC) or the corresponding cranial nerve motor nuclei with its axon. It forms the final common efferent pathway for any part of body.

There are two types of lower motor neurons namely the alpha and gamma motor neuron.

- The alpha motor neuron supplies extrafusal muscle fibres
- Gamma motor neuron supplies the contractile part (polar ends) of intrafusal muscle fibres.

Upper motor neuron (UMN) is any motor neuron which takes origin from the cerebral cortex or subcortical regions and influence the activity of lower motor neuron. All the descending tracts in general constitute the extensions of upper motor neuron in the spinal cord. They ultimately act on the lower motor neuron.

Differences between UMN and LMN lesions (Table 5.2 and Fig. 5.7)

Table 5.2 Differences between upper motor (UMN) and lower motor (LMN) neuron lesions

	UMN	LMN
Muscles affected	More in number	very few
Muscle tone	Increased (hypertonia)	lost (atonia)
Reflexes		
a. Superficial	All lost except plantar which is Babinski +ve	lost
b. Deep	Exaggerated	lost
Muscle wasting	Doesn't occur	yes (atrophy)
Type of paralysis	Spastic	flaccid
Reaction of degeneration	Absent	present
Site of lesion	Pyramidal or extra pyramidal tract lesion	Cranial or anterior nerve root lesion

Effect of dorsal/posterior/afferent nerve sectioning (Fig. 5.8)

Dorsal nerve carries all sensory input from the peripheral parts of body. It forms the afferent part of the basic reflex arc.

Features are *(in the affected part of the body)*

a. Loss of all sensations in a particular dermatome (if 3 consecutive nerve roots of the spinal cord are involved) due to damage in the afferent nerve fibres.

b. Loss of all reflexes due to lesion in the afferent part of basic reflex arc.

c. Tone of the muscle is lost due to damage in alpha gamma linkage pathway.

d. Voluntary movements are still present but not normal. This is because both the lower and upper motor neurons are intact but feed back signals from the concerned part are absent through the afferent nerve for co-ordination of movements.

e. Tissue damage and ulcers due to loss of protective pain sensations.

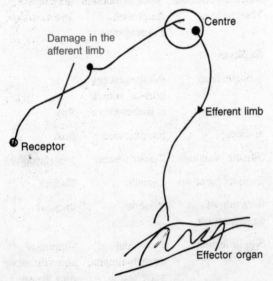

Fig. 5.8 Diagram showing lesion in afferent limb

Spinal Cord

In the vertebral column the extension of the CNS is nothing but spinal cord. It forms a connection between the brain and peripheral parts of body. There are 31 segments in spinal cord the division of segements are as follows:

- 8 cervical
- 12 thoracic
- 5 lumbar
- 5 sacral
- 1 coccygeal.

When a transverse section of spinal cord is looked at, in the inner part there is H shaped region with a canal (spinal canal) in the center. This part is called gray matter. The gray matter is composed of cell bodies of the neurons. The H shaped region is divisible into the anterior or ventral and posterior or dorsal horns. These horns are present in all the segments. Throughout the thoracic and in the upper segments of lumbar region, in addition to these horns there is lateral horn also. The afferent nerve enters the spinal cord through the posterior horn and the efferent nerve leaves the spinal cord through anterior horn.

Surrounding the gray matter region is the white matter. The white matter region can be divisible into 3 funiculi.

- Anterior funiculus-present between anterior nerve root and midline
- Lateral funiculus - present between posterior and anterior nerve roots
- Posterior funiculus-present between posterior nerve root and the midline

This region contains bundles of nerve fibres namely the tracts. Some of the tracts carry information from the spinal cord to higher parts of CNS and are known as ascending tracts.

Whereas the tracts which carry information from the higher parts of CNS to motor neuons of spinal cord are called as descending tracts. For proper functioning of the nervous system the impulse traffic through these tracts is very essential.

Tract, by definition, is the bundle of nerve fibers in CNS, which has common

- **Origin**
- **Course**
- **Termination and**
- **Functions.**

ASCENDING TRACTS

- They are in general sensory tracts.

- The impulses carried by these tracts help for the conscious perception of stimulus when it reaches cerebral cortex.

- Most of these fibers end in the sensory cortex of the cerebral region.

- Some of them do carry information to the other parts of brain namely cerebellum and the reticular formation of brain stem, and these will not come to conscious perception (non sensory inputs).

Some of the important ascending tracts are

a. Tract of Goll and Burdach (Fasciculus Gracilis and Cuneatus/posterior column tracts/dorsal column tracts).

b. Lateral spinothalamic tract

c. Anterior spinothalamic tract

d. Spinocerebellar tracts

Tract of Goll and Burdach (Fig. 5.9)

This tract is also known as posterior column tract or fasciculus gracilis and cuneatus. The sensations carried by the tract are

1. Fine touch
2. Tactile localization and discrimination
3. Pressure
4. Proprioception (sense of position and movement of joints)
5. Stereognosis
6. Vibration

Pathway from the peripheral parts of body to the CNS.

- Dorsal nerve root (1st order neuron) carry impulses from the receptors to spinal cord.

- These dorsal nerves enter the spinal cord through the posterior horn and fibres reach the posterior funiculus and ascend up as tract of Goll and Burdach.

- On reaching the brain stem, fibers synapse in the gracile and cuneate nuclei present in medulla oblongata.

- From here the 2nd order fibres take origin. About 80% of fibres ascend up as internal arcuate fibres.

- These fibres cross the midline in upper part of medulla oblongata and form the sensory decussation. These fibres while passing through the brain stem region give collaterals to the reticular formation present there.

- They reach the thalamus and synapse in ventro postero lateral (VPL) nucleus.

- From this nucleus the 3rd order fibers take origin.

- Pass through the posterior limb of internal capsule

- Reach the sensory cortex area no. 3, 1and 2 present in the postcentral gyrus (present in the parietal lobe) which is the center for perception of all general sensations.

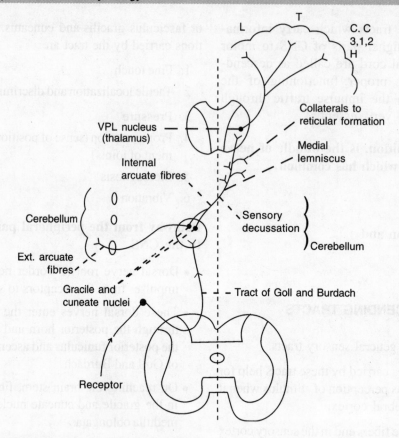

Fig. 5.9 Diagram showing the pathway of fine touch etc. from peripheral parts of body

Stereognosis

- Is the ability of the person to identify some familiar/known objects even with closed eyes
- The impulses for this will be carried by posterior column tracts
- The person is able to identify the object based on the
  - Shape
  - Size
  - Texture of the object.

Lateral spinothalamic tract (Fig. 5.10)

This tract carries the sensation of pain and temperature from the peripheral parts of body to the CNS.

- The fibres take origin from the receptors namely the free nerve endings.
- The fibres enter the spinal cord through the dorsal nerve root and synapse in subastantia gelatinosa Rolandi present in the posterior horn.
- From substantia gelatinosa the 2nd order fibres take origin, cross the midline in the anterior gray and white commisure to reach the lateral funiculus of the opposite side
- Ascend up as lateral spinothalmic tract. In the brainstem they give collaterals to the reticular formation.
- 2nd order fibres synapse in the ventro postero lateral nucleus of thalamus.

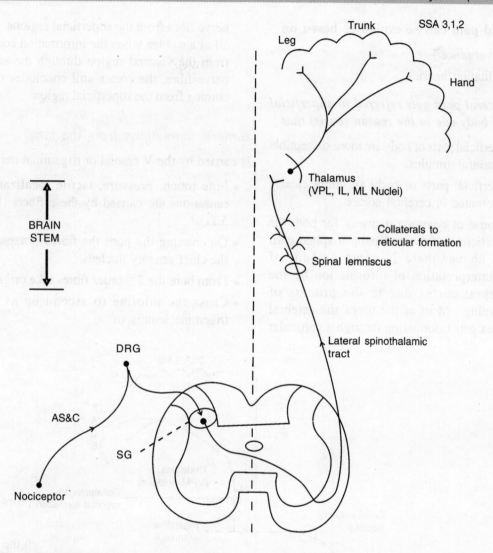

Fig. 5.10 Diagram showing the pathway of pain and temperature from peripheral parts of body

- From here the 3rd order fibres take origin, to reach cerebral cortex area no. 3, 1, and 2.
- Highest center for pain perception is thalamus.
- But fibers reaching the cortex help to
  a. Discriminate the intensity of pain
  b. Localize the area of pain more precisely
  c. Bring about an appropriate emotional reaction depending on the intensity of pain.

Referred pain

Pain in the viscera is normally not felt in the region of viscera but is referred to some superficial part of body which is away. Examples of referred pain are

- Heart pain is referred to left upper arm
- Appendicular pain is referred to umbilicus
- Tooth pain is referred to middle ear
- Diaphragmatic pain to tip of shoulder.

Referred pain can be explained based on

- Convergence
- Facilitation theories

The visceral pain gets referred to superficial parts of body due to the reason (basis) that

- Superficial parts of body are more susceptible for painful stimulus.
- Superficial parts of body are more clearly represented in cerebral cortex
- Because of common pathway for both the superficial and visceral pain in spinal cord and above, there is some amount of misinterpretation of information by the cerebral cortex due to the process of 'learning'. Most of the times the cerebral cortex gets information through a particular nerve fibre from the superficial regions and all of a sudden when the information comes from the visceral region through the same nerve fibre, the cortex still concludes it as coming from the superficial region.

General sensations from the face

Is carried by the V cranial or trigeminal nerve.

- Fine touch, pressure, tactile localization sensations are carried by these fibers (Fig. 5.11).
- On entering the pons the fibres synapse in the chief sensory nucleus.
- From here the 2nd order fibres take origin
- Cross the midline to ascend up as the trigeminal lemniscus

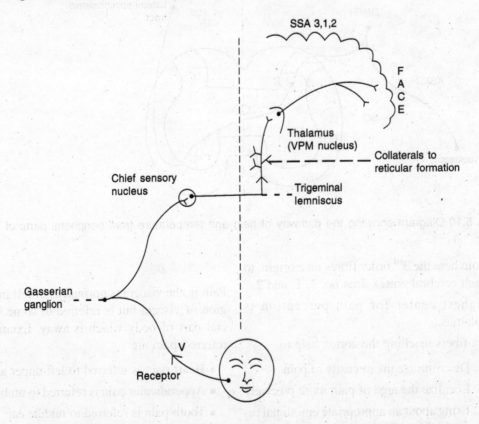

Fig. 5.11 Diagram showing the pathway for fine touch etc. from face region

- These fibres synapse in the ventro postero medial (VPM) nucleus of thalamus.
- From here the 3rd order fibres take origin pass through the posterior limb of internal capsule
- End in lateral most part regions of cerebral cortex area no. 3, 1 and 2.

Pain and temperature sensation from the face is also carried by the V cranial nerve (Fig. 5.12)

- From the receptors the fibres take origin

- Enter chief sensory nucleus region in pons
- *Fibres carrying pain sensation do not synapse in the chief sensory nucleus but merely pass through it.*
- Fibres carrying pain and temperature descend down in CNS to reach the upper parts of cervical segments of spinal cord and synapse in the spinal nucleus of V nerve.
- From here the 2nd order fibres take origin, cross the midline and ascend up as trigeminal lemniscus to reach thalamus.

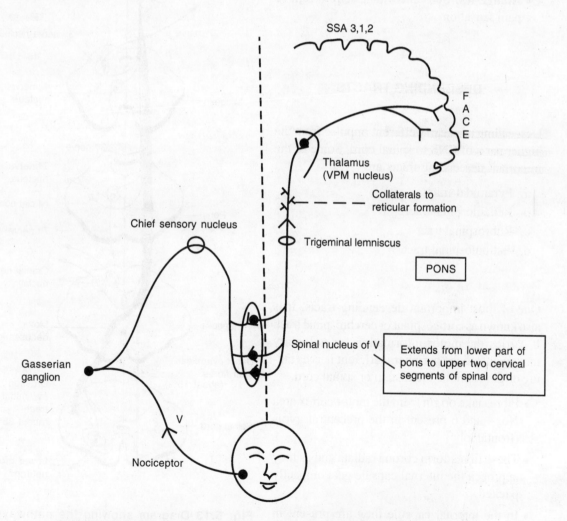

Fig. 5.12 Diagram showing the pathway for pain and temperature from face

- They also synapse in ventroposteromedial nucleus of thalamus.
- From this nucleus the 3rd order fibres take origin pass through the posterior limb of internal capsule
- End up in lateral most parts of cerebral cortex area No. 3, 1and 2.

General terminology

- **Anesthesia:** Loss of all sensations.
- **Analgesia:** Loss of pain sensation.
- **Analgesics:** Substances that help to relieve pain sensation.

DESCENDING TRACTS

Descending tract carry efferent impulse from the higher parts of CNS to spinal cord. Some of the important descending tracts are

a. Pyramidal tract
b. Reticulospinal tract
c. Rubrospinal tract
d. Vestibulospinal tract.

Pyramidal tract (Fig. 5.13)

One of most important descending tracts. It is also known as corticospinal or cerebrospinal tract. It carries the motor information for voluntary movements to the peripheral efferent nerves taking origin from the brain stem or spinal cord.

- Fibres take origin from the motor cortex area No. 4 and 6 present in the precentral gyrus (frontal lobe).
- These fibres form corona radiata and as they approach the internal capsule get compactly packed.
- In the internal capsule they are present in the anterior 2/3rd of posterior limb and genu.

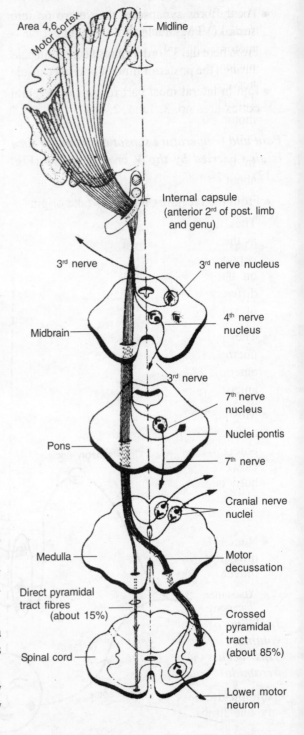

Fig. 5.13 Diagram showing the pathway of pyramidal tract

- As they descend down in the brain stem some of the fibres end on the cranial nerve motor nuclei of the opposite side. The nuclei on which these fibres end are cranial nerve nuclei of 3, 4, 5, 6, 7, 9, 10, 11 and 12. The fibres ending on cranial nerve motor nuclei of opposite side are called as cortico nuclear/cortico bulbar fibres.

- In the lower part of medulla oblongata about 85% of fibres cross the midline and form motor decussation.

- The fibres that have crossed are grouped as the lateral cortico spinal tract. This tract is present in the lateral funiculus. They end on the anterior horn cells present in the different segments throughout the length of spinal cord.

- The remaining 15% of fibres that are uncrossed run down in the spinal cord as anterior /ventral cortico spinal tract in the anterior funiculus.

- Most of these fibres cross the midline at different segments before ending on the anterior horn cells of opposite side. However some of them end on the anterior horn cells of the same side also.

Functions

- Necessary to perform all voluntary movements especially the skilled movements.
- Also helps to maintain muscle tone.

Inability of the person to bring about voluntary movements is known as paralysis. This occurs when there is lesion in the pyramidal tract.

Monoplegia: loss of voluntary movement in any one limb.

This occurs when there is involvement of lower motor neurons supplying any one limb.

Paraplegia: normally refers to the loss of voluntary movements in both the lower limbs.

This occurs when there is transversection of spinal cord above lumbosacral plexus.

Hemiplegia: generally means loss of voluntary movement in one half of body.

This occurs when there is lesion in internal capsule of one side.

Quadriplegia: loss of voluntary movements in all the parts of body except head and neck. All the 4 limbs of the body are paralysed.

This can occur when there is complete transection of spinal cord at the level of origin of brachial plexus (C6 segment of spinal cord).

Extrapyramidal tracts are also important for normal muscular activity and movement of various parts of body. The extrapyramidal tracts take origin from subcortical regions and brain stem.

Some of the important extrapyramidal tracts are-

1. Rubrospinal tract which takes origin from red nucleus in mid brain.

2. Reticulospinal tract which takes origin from reticular formation of brain stem.

3. Vestibulospinal which takes origin from vestibular nucleus in the brain stem.

The extrapyramidal tracts help to bring about normal movements by their influence on regulation of muscle tone which is very essential for normal activity.

Muscle tone gets affected in conditions like-

- Decerebrate rigidity
- Upper motor neuron lesions
- Parkinsonism
- Cerebellar lesion.

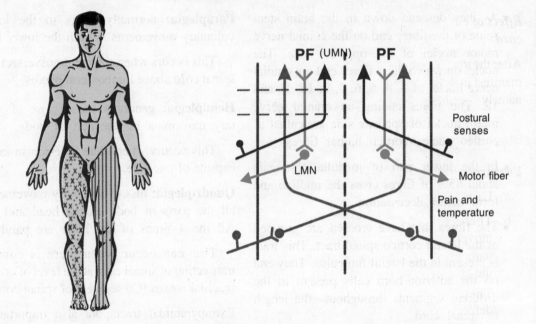

Fig. 5.14 Diagram showing effect of hemisection in spinal cord

Effect of hemisection of spinal cord (Fig. 5.14 and Table 5.3)

Dissociated anaesthesia means in a particular part of body certain sensation are lost and certain other sensations are present. For example in hemisection of spinal cord, below the level on the same side pain and temperature is intact and postural sensations are lost and vice versa on the opposite side. Dissociated anesthesia also occurs in syringomyelia, tabes dorsalis.

Table. 5.3 Effect of hemisection of spinal cord (Brown Sequard syndrome)

	On the same side	Opposite side
	Below the level of lesion	
Sensations		
Pain and temperature	Normal	Lost
Postural sensations	Lost	Normal
Motor functions	UMN lesion	Normal
	At the level of lesion	
Sensations	All sensations lost	Normal
Motor functions	LMN lesion	Normal
	Above the level of lesion	
Sensations	Hyperesthesia	Normal

Effect of complete transverse section of spinal cord

After the transection of the spinal cord the effects manifest in the affected parts of body in 3 stages namely

Stage of spinal shock

Features are

a. Lasts for about 6 weeks in human beings.

b. There will be no sensation, voluntary movements or reflexes (areflexia) in the parts affected, due to the damage to both the ascending and descending tracts.

c. There will be loss of micturition and defecations reflexes also.

d. Muscle tone will be lost completely (atonia).

e. Blood pressure gets decreased due to depression of the activity of the LHCs, if the lesion involves the upper 2 lumbar segments and above.

f. Skin will be cold and dry. Cyanosis may be seen.

All the features of spinal shock are due to the sudden withdrawl of supraspinal facilitatory influences to motor neurons of spinal cord. Because of this, the motor neuron undergo functional depression during the stage of spinal shock. They are able to recover the functional ability provided the shock period is ideally dealt with.

Taking care of patient during spinal shock stage

- Catheterization of the urinary bladder.
- Administering enema.
- Good nursing to prevent disuse atrophy and bed sores development.
- Proper antibiotics administration to take care of any infections.

Stage of recovery of reflex activity

During the stage of spinal shock, if proper care is taken, the affected part of the body gets into the next stage known as stage of recovery of reflex *activity. The recovery is because of the regaining of the functional ability of spinal cord neurons inspite of no influence from the higher centers.*

a. In this stage there will not be recovery of any voluntary movements or sensations as the damage to tracts is permanent.

b. *The spinal motor neurons (LHCs and AHCs) recover their functional ability, which enables the micturition and defecation reflexes* to become purely automatic.

c. Because of the recovery of LHC activity there will be regain of peripheral resistance and leads to increase of blood pressure though not to the normal level.

d. There will be recovery of muscle tone. Tone gets recovered earlier in the flexor compartment and later on in the extensor group of muscles. So flexion withdrawal reflex can be demonstrated now. Plantar reflex will be of Babinski +ve now. All the other superficial reflexes will be absent. When the muscle tone gets recovered in the extensor group of muscles, most of the times the lower limbs will be extended state. This is known as paraplegia in extension.

e. Deep reflexes of extensor group become exaggerated and clonic contractions appear.

f. Micturition and defecation become purely automatic.

Stage of reflex failure

- This is mainly because of infections.
- The toxins liberated by the bacteria may depress the activity of the motor neurons.
- There will be loss of muscle tone and all reflexes including micturition and defecation.
- Even the blood pressure falls.

CEREBELLUM

It is connected to the other parts of CNS through 3 pairs of peduncles namely superior, middle and inferior cerebellar peduncle. The afferent impulses that reach cerebellum don't come to conscious perception.

Functionally/physiologically cerebellum can be divisible into 3 parts:

Functionally into

a. Vestibulocerebellum (flocculonodular lobe)

b. Spinocerebellum (vermis and adjacent parts)

c. Cerebrocerebellum (lateral most parts of cerebellum).

Phylogenetically cerebellum is divided into

a. Archicerebellum

b. Paleocerebellum

c. Neocerebellum.

Some of the important afferent connections are

- Cuneo cerebellar fibres carry proprioceptive inputs from muscles of trunk and neck.

- Dorsal and ventral spino cerebellar tracts carry proprioceptive inputs from all parts of body.

- Vestibulo cerebellar tracts proprioceptive inputs from vestibular apparatus.

- Motor and premotor cortex as cortico ponto cerebellar fibres.

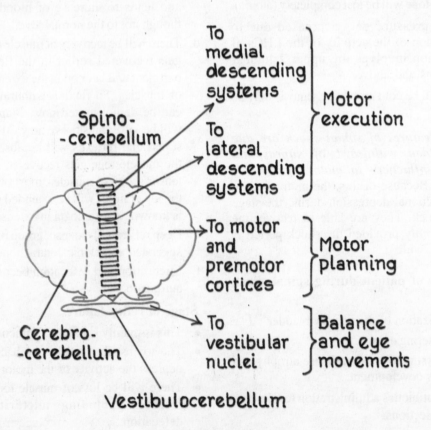

Fig. 5.15 Functional divisions of the cerebellum

Efferent connections are

- Cerebellovestibular from cerebellum to vestibular nucleus.
- Dentate rubrothalamocortical from dentate nucleus of cerebellum to red nucleus, thalamus and motor cortex.
- To the reticular formation of the brain stem from the emboliform, globose and fastigial nuclei.
- To the motor nuclei (3, 4 & 6) in the brain stem which supply the extraocular muscles.

Most of the efferent fibres from the cerebellum take origin from the 4 nuclei present in it. The nuclei are

a. Dentate
b. Emboliform
c. Globose
d. Fastigius.

Functions

1. Regulation of posture and equilibrium. The vestibulocerebellum performs this. Damage to this part will bring about postural imbalance and movements. It controls the activity of the axial and limb muscles. Inputs to cerebellum comes from the vestibular apparatus in the inner ear and from the receptors of muscles and joints also. Efferent output go to all the axial and limb muscles from the cerebellum through the vestibulo spinal and reticulo spinal tracts of the spinal cord.

2. Co-ordination of movements is brought about by involvement of cerebrocerebellum. It controls the activity of different set of muscles like agonist, antagonist and synergestic groups and help to bring about smooth movements in various joints. During the course of any movement there should be proper control over the rate, range, force and direction of movement. Co-ordination is possible because the cerebellum re-

ceives a copy of the motor command from motor areas and also constantly receives information about the performace in the different joints through many afferents. Cerebellum compares the motor command with that of movements getting executed and if there is any error, it will be informed to cerebral cortex. *Because of this cerebellum can act as a servocomparator.*

3. Regulation of automatic associated movements like swinging of the arms while walking.

4. Helps to regulate muscle tone by sending excitatory inputs to anterior horn cells in spinal cord either through the vestibular nucleus or through the reticular formation in the brain stem.

5. Regulates the movement of extraocular muscles and thereby able to keep the vision fixed on an object even when there is movement of head.

Some of the features of cerebellar lesion are:

a. Imbalance in posture and equilibrium
b. In co-ordination of movements (ataxia)
c. Kinetic or intention tremors
d. Slow scanning speech
e. Hypotonia
f. Nystagmus
g. Pendular knee jerk.

BASAL GANGLIA

Is one of the important parts in the subcortical region of brain. Composed of many nuclei namely caudate nucleus, putamen, globus pallidus, substantia nigra and subthalamic nucleus. Nuclei of basal ganglia and cerebral cortex have lot of closed circuit connections. Even between the nuclei there are a number of to and fro connections. The final efferent output from the nuclei

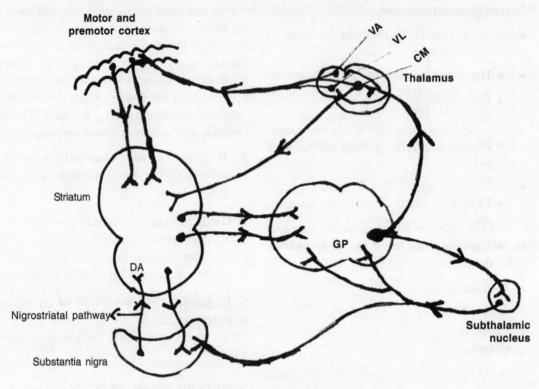

Fig. 5.16 Diagram showing basal ganglia connections

reach the motor and premotor cortex. This is the place from where the afferent inputs reach basal ganglia to start with.

Functions

a. Planning and programming of movements that is conversion of idea into an action.

b. Helps to bring about sub conscious movements like facial expressions, body language etc.

c. Provides postural background for any movement.

d. Regulation of muscle tone.

e. Primary motor cortex in lower animals in which there is no motor cortex.

Parkinsonism: *Is due to the lesion in the nigro-triatal pathway (dopamine is the neurotransmitter at this pathway) of basal ganglia.*

Some of the features are

- Hypertonia in all the muscles except in the extraocular muscles. Because of this it can lead to either lead pipe or cogwheel rigidity.

- Static/resting tremors especially the pill rolling movements. Tremors disappear during sleep.

- Akinesia or bradykinesia and it means there will be no initiative to bring about voluntary movements.

- Facial expressions are lost.

- Slow monotonous speech.

- Automatic associated movements are lost like swinging of arms while walking.

Treatment

Giving L dopa since dopamine can't cross blood-brain barrier. L dopa gets converted to dopamine in the basal ganglia region.

VESTIBULAR APPARATUS AND FUNCTIONS

- They are present in the inner ear.
- The semicircular canals, utricle and saccule form the vestibular apparatus.
- Receptors of semicircular canals are known as cristae ampullaris and that of utricle and saccule are called otolith organs.
- The receptors present in them act as mechanoceptors.
- The mechanoceptors get stimulated when there is acceleration or deceleration of the body and dorsi or ventri flexion of the head.

Connections

Afferent:

a. Afferent impulses from the vestibular apparatus are carried to CNS by the vestibular component of vestibulo cochlear nerve.

b. Afferent inputs also come from the floculo nodular lobe of cerebellum.

Efferent:

a. Vestibulospinal connects vestibular nucleus of brain stem with anterior horn cells in spinal cord.

b. Impulses also reach the cranial nerve motor nuclei of 3, 4 & 6 nerves.

Functions

a. Helps to regulate posture and equilibrium.

b. Helps to regulate muscle tone.

c. Helps to bring about the coordinated movements of eyeballs to keep the vision fixed even when the head is moving (vestibuloocular reflex).

Excessive stimulation of the apparatus causes

- **Dizziness**
- **Nausea**
- **vomiting.**

Sense of rotation of the surrounding objects (giddiness) is felt in vertigo.

THALAMUS

Is composed of various nuclei. They are broadly divisible into

a. Specific projection nuclei like ventero postero medial (VPM), ventero postero lateral (VPL) nuclei and lateral and medial geniculate bodies etc.

b. Non-specific nuclei like intra laminar, pulvinar and mid line nuclei.

Thalamus is strategically placed between cerebral cortex and the other parts of CNS. Hence most of the impulses either reaching cortex or from the cortex to reach other parts of CNS mostly relay in thalamic nuclei.

Afferent connections of thalamus

It forms relay station for almost all afferent inputs except olfaction. Some of the important afferent inputs to thalamus are impulses coming along

a. Tract of Goll and Burdach

b. Lateral and anterior spinothalamic tracts

c. Optic pathway

d. Auditory pathway

e. Trigeminal pathway

f. Taste pathway.

Efferent connections of thalamus

Most of the motor outputs going from the brain to reach the other parts of body get relayed in the nuclei of thalamus. Some of the important efferent connections are

a. Impulses coming from basal ganglia before reaching cerebral cortex
b. Impulses coming from dentate nucleus of cerebellum along the way to cerebral cortex
c. Impulses from the reticular formation of brain stem along the way to almost all parts of cerebral cortex.

Functions

a. Act as relay station for all sensory information except olfaction.
b. Act as relay station for motor output from cerebellum and basal ganglia to cerebral cortex.
c. It is the highest center for crude sensation

namely pain and temperature sensation including crude touch.

d. Concerned with short term memory.
e. Involved in emotional expressions.

HYPOTHALAMUS

This is one of the important subcortical regions. It has a number of nuclei. Some of the important nuclei are

- Supraoptic
- Paraventricular
- Lateral hypothalamic
- Ventromedial
- Preoptic
- Suprachiasmatic etc.

Table 5.4 Connections of hypothalamus

Tract	Type	Description
Medial forebrain bundle	A, E	Connects limbic lobe and midbrain via lateral hypothalamus
Fornix	A, E	Connects hippocampus to hypothalamus, mostly mamillary bodies
Stria terminalis	A	Connects amygdala to hypothalamus, mostly mamillary bodies
Mamillary peduncle	A	Connects brain stem to lateral mamillary nuclei
Dorsal noradrenergic bundle	A	Axons of noradrenergic neurons projecting from locus ceruleus to dorsal hypothalamus
Vascular Connection	E	Hypothalamo Hypophyseal Portal system connects hypothalamus with anterior pituitary gland
Retinohypothalamic fibers	A	Optic nerve fibers to suprachiasmatic nuclei from optic chiasm
Mamillothalamic tract of Vicq d'Azyr	E	Connects mamillary nuclei to anterior thalamic nuclei
Mamillotegmental tract	E	Connects hypothalamus to reticular portions of midbrain
Hypothalamohypophyseal tract	E	Axons of neurons in supraoptic and paraventricular nuclei

Some of the important connections (Table 5.4) **are** *with thalamus, limbic system, reticular formation through ascending reticular activating system, pituitary gland through the hypothlamo hypophyseal tract (neural connection with posterior pituitary gland only) and portal system (Vascular connection with anterior pituitary gland only)*

Functions

1. Thermoregulation is because of the involvement of heat loss and heat gain centers and also due to the activity of the preoptic nucleus, which acts as biologic thermostat. Anterior hypothalamic nucleus acts as heat loss center and posterior hypothalamic nucleus acts as heat gain center. Depending on the temperature of the body the altered activity of these centers bring about appropriate alterations in the activities in the body for restoration of the body temperature. Most of the influence is through the involvement of sympathetic nervous system.

2. Endocrine control is because of the hormone secretions from glands like pituitary, thyroid, adrenal cortex and gonads is due to the activity of hypothalamus. It can control secretions by acting through the pituitary gland. Hence hypothalamus has role in regulation of metabolism, growth and sexual activity. The anterior pituitary secretions are intimately regulated by the secretion of releasing hormone/factor or release inhibiting hormone/factor from the hypothalamus. The factors reach the anterior pituitary through the portal vessels.

3. Water metabolism is due to the secreting ability of ADH by the supraoptic nucleus and also due to the presence of thirst center in lateral hypothalamic nucleus. The osmoreceptors present in the hypothalamus also have a vital role to play in water metabolism and maintaining the osmolality of plasma.

4. Food intake regulation is due to the activity of satiety center present in ventro medial nucleus and the hunger center in lateral hypothalamic nucleus. If satiety center is damaged, the person keeps on eating (polyphagia). If hunger center is destroyed the person develops anorexia. Insulin is required for the glucose metabolism by the satiety center. When satiety center is active, it inhibits the activity of the hunger center. But the hunger center is a tonically active center and due to faulty glucose metabolism in diabetes mellitus, the inhibition by the satiety center on the hunger center is lost. This results in polyphagia.

5. Emotions: the bodily changes both somatic and autonomic during emotional reactions are associated with the functioning of the hypothalamus.

6. Autonomic nervous system (ANS): it is the highest center for ANS and hence can alter the activity of both the sympathetic and parasympathetic nervous system. Due to this there can be alteration in blood pressure, heart rate, gastro intestinal secretions, respiratory activity etc.

7. Biologic clock: suprachiasmatic nucleus acts as biologic clock and helps to keep track of *time in the body to bring about certain changes in the body functions according to the variations in time (diurnal variations).*

RETICULAR FORMATION

Deeply situated, ill-defined collection of nerve cells and their fibres with diffuse connections throughout the central part of brain stem. They are purely neural network pathways and have definite nuclear groups in the brainstem that act as centers to regulate the activity of many of the vital organs in our body. It has got extensive connection with many parts of central nervous system. Some of the connections are as per Fig. 5.17.

Some of the afferent connections are

a. From the spinal cord through collaterals of all the ascending tracts which carry general sensations. The general sensations from the face as well reach this area.

b. From the vestibular apparatus and pathways

c. Visual and auditory pathways also give collaterals including the taste pathway.

Some of the efferent connections are

1. Reticulo spinal tract connecting the reticular formation of brainstem with anterior and lateral horn cells in the spinal cord.

2. Connections are extended to cerebellum, red nucleus and tectum of mid brain.

3. Ascending reticular activating system (ARAS) reaching cerebral cortex via thalamus and hypothalamic nuclei.

Functions

1. Somatomotor function

Control of muscle tone through its connection with the anterior horn cells in the spinal cord. Predominantly it exerts inhibitory influence. The areas controlling the regulation of muscle tone are present in pons and medulla oblongata. The pontine influence is facilitatory whereas the bulbar (medullary) influence is inhibitory.

2. Viscero motor function

Regulation of most of the activities of visceral organs like heart, gastro intestinal tract, respiratory system. Hence it plays an important role in regulation of blood pressure, heart rate, respiration, gastro intestinal secretions and movements

This is possible because almost all the vital centers are present in the reticular formation of the brain stem.

3. Control of endocrine function

Regulates the secretion of most of the hormones

1. Motor and premotor cortex.
2. Basal ganglia
3. Cerebellum
4. Lnhibitory reticular formation
5. Facilitatory reticular formation.
6. Vestibular nucleus.

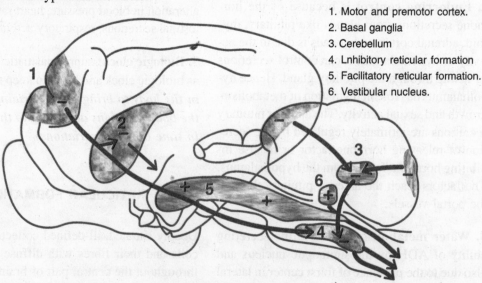

Fig. 5.17 Some of the connections of reticular formation

in the body and hence it influences almost all metabolisms. It is due to the involvement of hypothalamus, which is considered to be master endocrine gland. The hypothalamic secretions are essential for most of the hormonal secretions in our body.

4. Ascending reticular activating system: Help in sleep, arousal and alert state of the individual because of the efferent connection with the cerebral cortex through the hypothalamus.

5. Somatosensory functions
Almost all the sensory inputs are fed to reticular formation through collaterals along their course to cerebral cortex. Hence this helps for modulation of sensory inputs by descending pathways acting on the spinal cord. It is also involved in alert reaction of the individual due to ARAS.

CEREBRO SPINAL FLUID (CSF)

- It is a special fluid present in the ventricles of brain, central canal of spinal cord, subarachnoid spaces and interstitium of CNS.
- The choroid plexus present in the lateral, third & fourth ventricles secrete it.
- It gets absorbed through the archnoid villi into the subdural venous sinuses.
- The normal volume is about 150 ml and daily turn over is about 500 ml.
- **Some of the important constituents of CSF are**
  - **K^+**   **3 mEq/kg water**
  - **Ca^{++}**   **2.5 mEq/kg water**
  - **Cl^-**   **110 mEq/kg water**
  - **Glucose 60 mg%**
  - **Proteins 40 mg%.**

The concentration of these substance will not be same **as in plasma.**

- Normal pressure is about 130 mm CSF.

Functions

1. Protection of the brain against mechanical trauma as it can act as shock absorber.

2. Acts as a medium for exchange of substances between neurons and blood. Helps to supply nutrition and oxygen to brain and removal of metabolic wastes carbon dioxide from nerves to blood.

3. Helps to maintain the contents of intracranial cavity constant by bringing about appropriate variations in the cerebro spinal fluid volume. If size of brain or volume of blood in cranial cavity is increased, the volume of cerebro- spinal fluid decreases proportionately.

4. Provides buoyancy effect to brain and hence the effective weight of the brain is reduced from 1500 g to 50 g. This helps for easy movement of head.

Lumbar puncture

Is a procedure in which special needle is introduced between L_3 and L_4 vertebrae into the subarachnoid spaces of spinal cord from the posterior aspect.

Significance

- To obtain a sample of cerebro spinal fluid for physical, chemical and microscopic examinations.
- To measure the intracranial tension.
- To introduce drugs which are unable cross blood brain barrier.
- To induce spinal anesthesia.

Blood-brain barrier

- Is formed by the tight junctions of capillary endothelium.

- The foot process of astrocytes also contribute for the development of barrier.

- This limits the movement of substances from blood into the brain.

- It is not developed completely at birth.

- There are certain parts of brain, which are devoid of blood brain barrier. These parts are neurohypophysis, subfornical organ, area postrema and organum vasculosum of lamina terminalis.

Functions

- Helps to maintain the constancy of the microenvironment around the neurons in CNS.

- Protection of neurons from toxic substances present in blood.

- Undue dispersal of chemical substances like neurotransmitter from getting escaped into the general circulation is prevented.

Importance

While administering certain substance in diseases of brain one should have the knowledge whether the substance can cross the barrier. Drugs like antibiotics can't cross the barrier when given orally or intravenously. In such a situation an alternate route of administration has to be looked into and it can be through lumbar puncture.

LIMBIC SYSTEM

Groups of cortical and subcortical structures arranged in a limbus (ring) around the hilum of cerebral hemisphere.

Components are

- Hippocampus
- Hypothalamus

- Cingulate gyrus
- Amygdala etc

Functions

1. Emotion: The various behavioral changes observed in conditions like rage, sex drive and pleasure are under the control of the activity of this region. Also plays a role in the control of emotions like fear, anxiety etc.

2. Autonomic changes like alterations in hormonal secretions, activity of ANS is controlled.

3. Motivation: Which helps the organism to perform certain tasks by which reward may be obtained or punishment is avoided.

4. Memory: Along with the hypothalamus it has an important role in consolidation of memory.

5. Parental behavior is affected when there is lesion in cingulate gyrus.

ELECTROENCEPHALOGRAM (EEG)

It is the graphical recording of the electrical activity of the cortical and subcortical structures. It can be recorded by placing the surface electrodes on the scalp region.

The different rhythms/waves are

a. **Alpha rhythm** is observed when the person is in awake state with mind wandering and eyes closed.

   The frequency and amplitude will be moderate.

   When eyes are opened or even with closed eyes if certain mental task like solving some mathematical problem is done, alpha waves are replaced by fast, low amplitude irregular waves. This is known as alpha block.

b. **Beta rhythm recording** is observed when the brain is in alert state. The frequency of the wave is high and amplitude is least.

c. **Theta rhythm** has larger amplitude. Sometimes seen in small children. They are also observed in adult when a person initiates motor activity in response to a stimulus.

d. **Delta rhythm** has least frequency and maximum amplitude. It is recorded during NREM sleep (NREM–non rapid eye movement).

Significance of EEG recording

- Foci of epilepsy can be identified.
- Alterations in the recording can be seen in brain tumors, cerebral hemorrhage and precise site of problems can also be made out.
- To ascertain whether the patient is brain dead in coma stage.

Sleep

Is a state of temporary unconsciousness from which a person can be easily aroused. There are two different types of sleep. NREM (Non-REM) and REM (rapid eye movement) sleep.

NREM sleep features

1. No movement of eyeballs.
2. Muscle tone is reduced.
3. Cardiovascular and respiratory functions are more stable and least.
4. Theta and delta rhythm EEG pattern is observed.

REM sleep features

1. EEG resembles the one recorded during the alert state.
2. Person is in deep sleep.
3. Rapid eye movement occur.

4. Person experiences dreams.
5. Irregularity in heart rate, blood pressure and respirations.
6. There can be penile erection and at times ejaculations as well.

FUNCTIONAL AREAS OF CEREBRAL CORTEX (Fig. 5.18)

1. **Sensory area is** present in postcentral gyrus area No. 3, 1 & 2. All the general sensory pathways from the peripheral parts of body end here. It is the centre for all general sensations and also for taste.

   The body is represented upside down and contralaterally in the homunculus way. The extent of representation of the different parts of body in this region depends on the density of the receptors in the concerned part of body.

2. **Motor area is** present in precentral gyrus area No 4 and 6. Pyramidal tract fibres take origin from this region.

   The body representation is contra lateral and upside down. In this region it is not the individual muscles that are represented but the movements, which involve group of muscles. Initiates movements especially the skilled one (voluntary) in the opposite half of body and also helps in the regulation of muscle tone.

3. **Occipital lobe is** the center of vision. The area Nos. is 17, 18 and 19. Area 17 acts as primary area and area 18 & 19 act as association area for vision. The visual pathway ends in this region.

4. **Auditory area will** be area No. 41, 42 (primary auditory area) and No. 21and 22

(auditory association area). They are present in auditory cortex in the temporal lobe. The auditory pathway fibres end here. They help for perception of sound and also the analysis of the sound heard.

5. **Frontal eye field** is present in frontal cortex area No. 8. It is responsible for the conjugated eye movements while following an object.

6. *Broca's area of speech is area no.44. It is present in the dominant hemisphere and controls all voluntary speech.*

LEARNING AND MEMORY

Learning

- Is change in behavior based on the past experience for the stimulus.

- There are two types of learning namely associative and non associative learning.
- Associative learning can be classical or instrumental conditioning as demonstrated by Pavlov.
- In non-associative learning the organism learns about a single stimulus.

Memory

- Is the ability of the organism to register, retain and recall the information at a later date.

- The different types of memory are short and long term.

- Short-term memory is not stored permanently e.g. recalling of some phone number for a short duration after scanning the directory.

- Long term is one where recalling ability lasts for months and years like the name and place

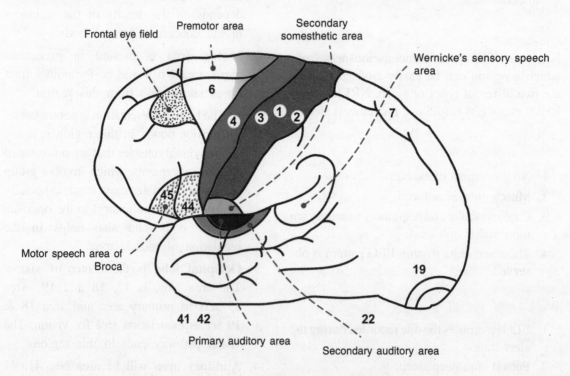

Fig. 5.18 Some of the important areas of cerebral cortex

of school one has studied, the native place of a person etc.

Amnesia is inability of the person to recall the information. There are two types of amnesia namely anterograde and retrograde. Retrograde amnesia is when there is inability to recall the memory stored earlier to the incident. In anterograde amnesia the ability to process the new information for consolidation of the memory is lost.

AUTONOMIC NERVOUS SYSTEM (ANS)

Part of the nervous system, which regulates the functioning of the visceral organs. The two different limbs of autonomic nervous system are sympathetic and parasympathetic.

Sympathetic takes origin from the lateral horn cells of the thoraco lumbar segments of spinal cord *whereas the parasympathetic* is from the cranial (in the brain) and sacral (in the spinal cord) regions. In the parasympathetic component the nerves included are cranial nerve 3, 7, 9 and 10 and also the pelvic nerve from the sacral segments of spinal cord.

- **Centers for autonomic nervous system are** *present in hypothalamus.*

- *The anterior hypothalamus controls the activity of parasympathetic and posterior hypothalamus the sympathetic parts.*

- *In any autonomic nervous system pathway there are two neurons along the efferent pathway. The preganglionic and postganglionic. The neurotransmitter at the pre and post ganglionic regions in parasympathetic part is acetylcholine. In sympathetic at preganglionic region*

it is acetylcholine whereas in the post-ganglionic region in most of the parts it is noradrenaline.

- *Acetylcholine can act through the nicotinic or muscarinic receptors present in the pre and post ganglionic regions respectively.*

- *Noradrenaline can act through the alpha or beta receptors.*

Functions of autonomic nervous system

1. Regulation of functions of visceral organs like heart, gastro intestinal tract etc and thereby help to regulate heart rate, blood pressure and gastro intestinal secretion and motility.

2. In lungs brings about bronco dilation when acts through sympathetic nerve and vice versa effect when the parasympathetic nerve stimulation is there.

3. Sweat glands are supplied by sympathetic cholinergic fibres and are involved in regulation of body temperature.

4. Secretions from the adrenal medulla are regulated by the activity of the sympathetic nerves (pelvic splanchnic nerve).

5. In eyes, the pupillary dilation is by sympathetic nerve stimulation and constriction by parasympathetic nerve stimulation.

6. Defecation and micturition will be brought about due to the activity of the parasympathetic nerves stimulation.

7. In male reproductive system errection of penis is due to parasympathetic stimulation and ejaculation is because of sympathetic nerve activity.

Nerve Muscle Physiology

- Introduction
- Neuron
- Action potential
- Nerve injuries
- Muscle
- Neuromuscular connection
- Excitation contraction coupling
- Rigor mortis
- Smooth muscle

INTRODUCTION

Function of the nervous system is to receive (receptive), analyse and transmit (conduct) the information.

Cells of the nervous system are classified into two types namely neurons and glial cells. Neurons are excitable and glial cells are non-excitable.

The glial cells are microglia, oligodendroglia and astrocytes.

a. Microglia are scavenger cells resembling the tissue macrophages.

b. Oligodendroglia are concerned with providing the myelin sheath to the nerve fibres in the central nervous system.

c. Astrocytes are of two types namely fibrous and protoplasmic astrocytes. Fibrous are found in the white matter and protoplasmic in the gray matter. Both the types send process to the blood vessels in central nervous system to form tight junctions that form the blood brain barrier.

When compared to the neurons, the size of the glial cells is much less. The number of glial cell is about 10 to 50 times the number of neurons.

Some of the important definitions

Neuron—is the structural and functional unit of nervous system.

Nerve—collection of nerve fibres (axons) outside the central nervous system.

Ganglion—collection of nerve cell bodies outside the central nervous system.

Nucleus—collection of nerve cell bodies inside the central nervous system.

Centre—group of nerve cell bodies inside the central nervous system having common function.

Synapse—is functional junction between parts of two different neurons.

NEURON

It is a structural and functional unit of nervous system. Any neuron is made up of 3 parts namely axon (nerve fibre), cell body or soma and dendrites.

Classification of neurons can be done in different ways based on different criteria

Based on the structure the neurons can be classified into unipolar, bipolar and multipolar neurons (Fig. 6.1). In unipolar both the dendrites and axon take origin from the same pole. In bipolar they take origin from two different poles.

Based on function the neurons can be classified into sensory (afferent) or motor (efferent).

Based on the type of neurotransmitter released from the terminals of the axon e.*g*.

1. Cholinergic—acetylcholine (ACh)

2. Adrenergic—noradrenaline

3. Serotonergic—serotonin as the neurotransmitter etc.

Cell body and dendrites are the receiving parts of any neuron. The axon or nerve fibre does the conduction of impulse across long distance. The endings of the axon are branched and they are called as axon telodendria or terminal boutons.

Based on the histology, the nerve fibres are

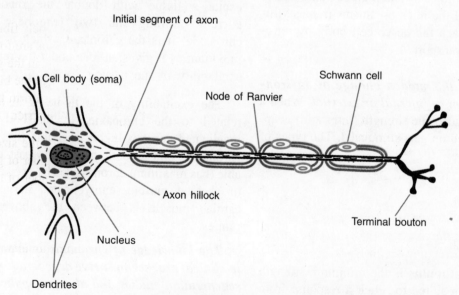

Fig 6.1 Diagram of a multipolar neuron

classified into two types namely unmyelinated and myelinated.

a. In a myelinated nerve fibre the sheath of Schwann cell (myelin sheath) covers the axon unlike the unmyelinated nerve fibre in which the Schwann cell just encircles the axon.

b. In a myelinated nerve fibre the myelin sheath is absent at certain places, which are known as nodes of Ranvier.

c. The presence of myelin sheath enhances the rate of conduction of the impulse. In the case of human beings it can be as fast as 70–120 m/sec.

The protoplasm that is present in the axon is known as axoplasm. The transport of substance through the axoplasmic flow can occur in any direction.

1. When the transport is from the cell body towards the axon terminal it is called anterograde and when it is in the opposite direction is known as retrograde transport.

2. The neurotransmitter substance reaches the axon terminal by anterograde transport and some of the microorganisms (rabies virus etc.) reach the nerve cell body by retrograde transport.

Stimulus *is the sudden change of environment that can be internal or external.* When a stimulus of adequate strength (threshold) is applied, the neuron gets stimulated. The types of stimuli can be

• Mechanical
• Chemical
• Thermal
• Electrical.

Threshold stimulus is the minimum strength of stimulus required to elicit a response from excitable tissue.

Excitation is the response obtained from any excitable tissue consequent to application of threshold stimulus and above. The excitation can be either an electrical change only (as in neuron) or both electrical and mechanical changes (as in muscle). There can also be thermal and chemical changes in the muscles.

The properties of the nerve are

a. *excitability*
b. *conductivity*
c. *refractory period and*
d. *all or none law.*

A. Excitability in the nerve gets manifested in the form of electrical change only. The electrical change leads to generation of an action potential (impulse) from the resting state (resting membrane potential) of the nerve.

Rheobase—is the minimum strength of stimulus required to stimulate (excite) a tissue without considering the time duration for which the stimulus has to be applied.

Chronaxie—is the minimum time required to excite a tissue with double the rheobasic current. Among the two (rheobase and chronaxie) it is the chronaxie, which is more important as it gives an idea about the relative excitability of the tissue.

The excitability of the tissue is inversely related to the chronaxie. In the body the myelinated nerve is highly excitable (has least chronaxie) and smooth muscle is least excitable (has maximum chronaxie). The excitability of skeletal muscle, unmyelinated nerve and cardiac muscle is between the above two ranges.

The knowledge of chronaxie is important in clinical practice for nerve degeneration and regeneration studies and also for application of the principle of diathermy.

Some of the factors, which can affect the excitability of the tissues, are:

- *Temperature*
- *Ionic composition especially calcium, sodium and potassium*
- *Local anesthetics*

B. Conductivity: Ability of the tissue to transmit the impulse from one end to the other (nerve fibre) . Even though the impulse gets transmitted for a long distance, the amplitude (height) of the action potential does not get decreased. This type of conduction is known as decrementless conduction.

As stated earlier one of the important factors, which affect the velocity of impulse conduction in nerve fibres is whether the nerve fibre is myelinated. In a myelinated nerve fibre the impulse jumps from one node of Ranvier to the next node. This type of conduction is called as saltatory or leaping conduction (Fig. 6.2).

Apart from the above some of the other factors, which can affect the velocity of impulse conduction, are

a. Diameter of nerve fibre

b. Pressure

c. Local anesthetics

d. Diseases (multiple sclerosis)

e. Temperature.

Based on the diameter and conduction velocity, the nerve fibres are classified into different types by Gasser and Erlanger. The three major types are A, B and C group fibres. The A group is further divided into alpha, beta, gamma and delta. The C group is divisible into dorsal root and sympathetics. A alpha type has maximum diameter and conduction velocity (70–120 m/sec) and C group has least diameter and conduction velocity (0.7–2.3 m/sec). The diameter and conduction velocity of the other groups are between the aforesaid ranges in decreasing order (Table 6.1).

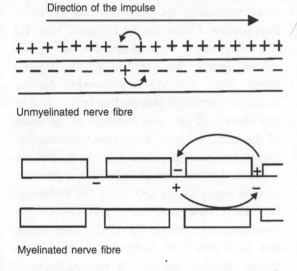

Direction of the impulse

Unmyelinated nerve fibre

Myelinated nerve fibre

Fig. 6.2 Impulse conduction in unmyelinated and myelinated nerve fibre

Table 6.1 Gasser and Erlanger classification

Fiber Type	Function	Fiber Diameter (µm)	Conduction velocity (m/s)
A			
α	Proprioception; somatic motor	12-20	70-120
β	Touch, pressure	5-12	30-70
γ	Motor to muscle spindles	3-6	15-30
δ	Pain, cold touch	2-5	12-30
B	Preganglionic autonomic	<3	3-15
C Dorsal root	Pain, temperature, some mechanoception reflex responses	0.4-1.2	0.5-2
Sympathetic	Post ganglionic sympathetics	0.3-1.3	0.7-2.3

A and B fibers are myelinated,
C fibers are unmyelinated

Susceptibility of the nerve fibres for failure to conduct impulse differs with the type of the factors.

- *For pressure it is the A group which is highly susceptible*
- *For hypoxia it is B group which is highly susceptible*
- *For local anesthetics it is C group which is highly susceptible.*

C. Refractory period is the duration after an effective stimulus when a second stimulus is applied there will not be response for the 2nd stimulus. It extends upto 1/3rd of repolarisation phase.

D. All or none law: When a tissue is stimulated either it responds maximally or not at all. For a stimulus strength of less than threshold (sub threshold) there will not be any response. For any threshold stimulus there is response which is maximum and hence for more than threshold stimulus (supra threshold) the amplitude of response shall remain the same. Tissues, which obey all or none law, are

a. **Single nerve fibre**

b. **Single skeletal muscle fibre**

c. **Cardiac muscle**

d. **A motor unit**

e. **Visceral smooth muscle**

f. **Single fibre of multiunit smooth muscle.**

Resting membrane potential (RMP)

Resting membrane potential (RMP) is the potential difference that exists between the extracellular fluid (ECF) and intracellular fluid regions (ICF) (that is across the cell membrane) when the tissue is at rest. Normally when compared to extracellular fluid, the intracellular fluid part is negative. Hence the resting membrane potential value is always is prefixed with a -ve symbol.

Resting membrane potential varies with the tissues. In a nerve fibre it is mostly around -70 mV.

Resting membrane potential is always due to the unequal distribution of the charged substances in extracellular and intracellular fluid regions. Some of the important charged ions distribution in the regions are as follows:

Substance	ECF	ICF
Na$^+$	150 mEq/L	15 mEq/L
K$^+$	5 mEq/L	150 mEq/L
Cl$^-$	105 meq/L	10 meq/L
Organic anions (− charged)	Not much	A lot

Sodium tries to move (diffuse) into intracellular fluid along the electrochemical gradient, potassium tries to move out into extra cellular fluid along concentration gradient only and chloride tries to move in along concentration gradient alone. The cell membrane is more permeable for potassium ion diffusion than sodium. Unlike for the inorganic ions, the cell membrane is impermeable for the organic anions. Hence the retention of the organic anions inside the cell is responsible for the negative membrane potential at rest. Even at rest there will be some amount of diffusion of the inorganic ions along either the concentration or electrical gradient or both. But the restoration of the ions at respective regions is brought about by the activity of the pump e.g. Na$^+$-K$^+$ ATPase pump which removes sodium from intra cellular to extra cellular fluid region and vice versa for potassium, which keep getting diffused because of the gradients.

When a stimulus of threshold intensity or above is applied, the polarity of the membrane is altered. The intracellular fluid part, which is normally negative, now becomes positive. This type of reversal of the polarity of the membrane is known as depolarization.

After a few milliseconds, the polarity of the membrane gets reestablished (intracellular fluid again becomes negative). This is known as repolarisation. When the membrane potential becomes more negative it is called hyperpolarisation and when it becomes less negative it is hypopolarisation (depolarisation).

When hypopolarising (depolarising) type of current is developed and is of sufficient value (reaching firing level) it brings about the development of action potential.

Application of sub threshold stimulus makes the membrane less negative (hypopolarising) but since it is not reaching the firing level there will not be production of action potential. There will be production of only the local potential. The amplitude of local potential is dependent on the strength of stimulus and the duration of local potential is more when compared to the action potential. Unlike action potential that is all or none in nature, the local potentials can be summated by application of a number of sub threshold stimuli (Table 6.2).

Local potentials get produced at different places like at

- *Receptor—receptor potential*
- **Neuro muscular junction —end plate potential (EPP)**
- *Synapse—excitatory or inhibitory post synaptic potential (EPSP/IPSP).*

ACTION POTENTIAL

Is a brief, propagated depolarization process which can get conducted a long distance on application of threshold stimulus. The action poten-

Differences between	Local potential	Action potential
Size	graded	all or none
Conduction	not well (Decrementing type)	decrementless
Summation	Possible	Not possible
Polarity	depolarizing or hyperpolarizing type	always depola-ing type
Intensity of stimulus	Not fixed	Threshold and above
Refractory period	Nil	Present
Function served	Signal over short distances	Signal over long distances

Table 6.2 Differences between action potential and local potential

tial while getting conducted keeps self-regenerating.

During the action potential development the membrane of the tissue becomes permeable for sodium. So the sodium ions move from the extra cellular fluid into the intracellular fluid region. Because of the influx of the sodium ions, the interior becomes positive as against the negative state observed during the resting condition. The reversal of polarity due to sudden influx of sodium ions is responsible for the process of depolarization. The sodium ion flux is so much that the membrane potential exceeds the zero potential and over shoots. The potential reachs as much as + 35 mV (Fig.6.3 and the schematic diagram of monophasic action potential and ionic basis for the same has been shown in Fig. 6.4)

During the later part of depolarization the sodium channels begin to close and potassium

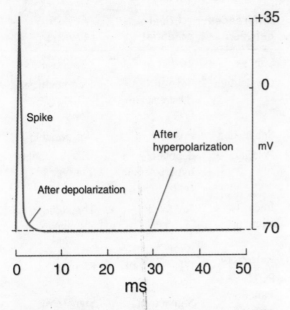

Fig. 6.3 Actual recording of monophasic action potential

channels start opening up. Because of this there will be efflux of potassium ions. The outward movement of potassium ions will bring about the reestablishment of polarized state (repolarisation) of the membrane.

The amplitude and configuration of the action potential varies with the tissue. The diagram above is specifically of the action potential (monophasic) recorded from a nerve fibre.

Types of action potential

From a single nerve fibre or a muscle fibre we can record either *a monophasic or biphasic action potential.* For recording a monophasic action potential recording one of the recording electrodes should be in extracellular and the other electrode in the intracelluar fluid regions. For biphasic action potential recording, both the recording electrodes may be kept either in intracellular or extracellular fluid regions. The action potential can be recorded on a CRO (cathode ray oscilloscope).

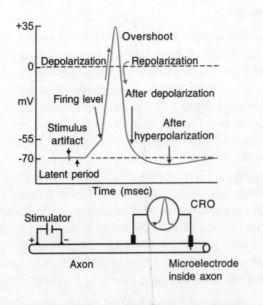

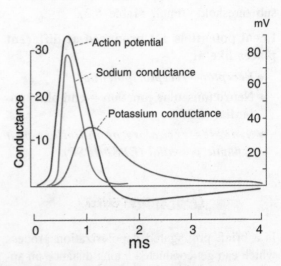

Fig 6.4 Schematic diagram of monophasic action potential with ionic conductance

Compound action potential is summated action potential that can be recorded from a mixed nerve. Mixed nerve means it can have some nerve fibres that are afferent, and some that are efferent.

A mixed nerve can also be purely afferent or efferent but has nerve fibres belonging to different groups according to the Gasser and Erlanger's classification. Compound action potential will have many peaks and the peaks appear at different times because of variation in conduction velocity. The amplitude of the peak is dependent on the presence of number of nerve fibres belonging to a particular group.

An impulse can get conducted in either direction. When it gets conducted in the usual direction (in afferent it is towards central nervous system and vice versa in efferent) it is known as orthodromic conduction. If the conduction of impulse in the nerve fibre is against the usual direction of conduction, it is known as antidromic conduction.

As stated the action potential once generated, by itself can't get conducted during the course of conduction. The local currents developed in the adjacent region bring about the development of another action potential having the same amplitude. Hence it is termed as self-regenerating type and gets conducted in decrementless fashion.

NERVE INJURIES

a. Neurapraxia is physiological paralysis. Conduction of impulse in the intact nerve fibres suffers due to application of pressure without any rupture. There will be no degeneration of the nerve fibres.

b. Axonotemesis is when nerve fibres get ruptured within an intact endoneurial tube. There will be degeneration of nerve fibres.

c. Neuranotemesis is partial or complete division of nerve sheath and fibres. There will be degeneration of the nerve fibres.

Degeneration

When there is damage to the nerve fibres the degenerative changes seen are

a. Changes in the distal segment of axon

- Axon breaking up into small cylindrical structures, myelin sheath breaks up into oil droplets

- Debris fills up the endoneurial tube

- Macrophages clear the debris.

b. In the proximal part of the axon also all the above changes can be observed. In general these changes are included under Wallerian degeneration.

c. Changes in the cell body will be

- Disintegration of Nissl substance and there will be chromatolysis.

- The nucleus might be pushed to a side and at times it may be lost.

All the above changes are histological changes.

The physiologic change observed depends on whether the nerve fibres damaged are sensory or motor in function.

- In case the the degenerated nerve is sensory there will be loss of sensations in the affected parts of the body.

- If degenerated nerve is motor in function, it leads to paralysis in the affected part of the body.

- Now to stimulate the muscle stimulus has to be sent for more duration than it used to be when the nerve supply was intact.

Regeneration

The regenerative changes will be

a. Multiplication of Schwann cells to bridge the gap between the cut ends, that is between the proximal and distal parts of the endoneurial tube.

b. Axon shows multiple sprouting of fibrils from the proximal end, but only one of the fibrils succeeds in reaching the distal part. After this has taken place, the other fibrils get degenerated and the one that has reached the distal part continues to grow. The rate of growth of the nerve fibre will be about 1 mm/day.

c. Schwann cells contribute for the myelin sheath around the regenerative nerve fibre. Regeneration of the nerve fibre is complete only after proper myelination.

Factors influencing the regeneration are

a. Gap between the cut ends when less than 3 mm, regeneration can occur.

b. Suturing of the nerve trunk will speed up the regeneration.

c. The gap should not be filled by any other fluid or tissue or foreign object.

d. The infections should be avoided at the site of injury.

e. If the injury is closer to the cell body the neuron dies. So regeneration will not be possible.

f. Age of the person.

MUSCLE

Muscles in the body are in general required for movements and stability. They are also excitable tissues like neuron.

Classification of the muscles in the body can be done in different ways.

a. Based on the whether there are definite cross striations in the muscle fibre, they can be classified into striated and non-striated muscle.

b. Based on whether the muscles are under voluntary control, they can be classified into voluntary and involuntary muscle.

c. Based on location they can be classified into skeletal, cardiac and smooth muscle.

Skeletal muscles are voluntary and striated, cardiac muscle is involuntary and striated and smooth muscles are involuntary and non-striated (Table 6.3).

Table 6.3 Characteristic features of skeletal, cardiac and smooth muscle

Characteristics	Skeletal	Smooth	Cardiac
Properties			
1. Rhythmicity	Absent	Present	Present
2. Conductivity	Very fast	Slow	Slow
3. All-or-none law	Single fibre	Present	Present (whole heart)
Distribution	Skeletal	Hollow viscera	Only heart
Control	Voluntary	Involuntary	Involuntary
Nerve supply	Somatic	Autonomic	Autonomic

Skeletal muscle

Sarcomere (Fig. 6.5) is the structural and functional unit of muscle fibre. It includes the structures present between two consecutive Z lines.

- 'A' band is made up of myosin protein.
- 'I' band is made up of actin, tropomyosin and troponin proteins.
- The actin and myosin are known as contractile proteins and troponin and tropomyosin are regulatory proteins.
- The invaginations of sarcolemma of the muscle fibres at the junction of A and I bands is called T (transverse) tubule.
- The sarcoplasmic reticulum (L tubule) placed horizontally between the T tubules and the terminal parts of it are dilated. These are called the lateral cisterns.
- Two lateral cisterns with one T tubule form sarcoplasmic triad.
- T tubule helps to conduct the impulse inside the muscle fibre and the cisterns store and release the calcium ions required for muscle contraction.

NEURO MUSCULAR JUNCTION

Neuromuscular junction is the functional junction between the ending of the motor neuron and muscle. For all practical purposes the muscle part that is normally considered is the skeletal muscle region (Figs. 6.6 and 6.7).

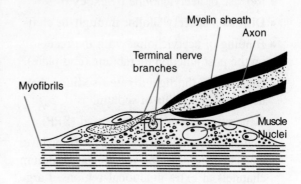

Fig 6.6 Diagram of neuromuscular junction

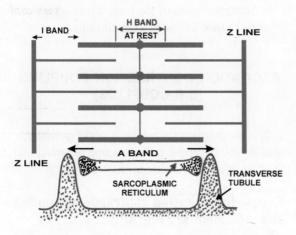

Fig. 6.5 Diagram of a sarcomere

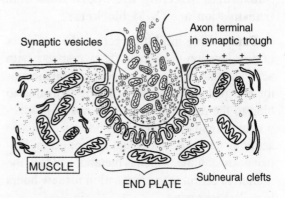

Fig 6.7 Diagram of neuromuscular junction (magnified view)

Steps in neuromuscular transmission

- Arrival of action potential (AP) at the motor neuron terminal.
- Depolarization of motor neuron terminal.
- Calcium ion influx into nerve terminals.
- Binding of synaptic vesicles to pre junctional membrane.
- Release of acetylcholine by exocytosis.
- Diffusion of acetylcholine through the clefts.
- Binding of acetylcholine with the receptors on the post junction membrane (end plate).
- Opening of the ligand gated sodium channels and slow influx of sodium.
- Generation of end plate potential (EPP).
- End plate potential on reaching the firing level leads to opening of the voltage gated sodium channels at extra junctional regions. Large influx of sodium.
- Generation of muscle action potential.
- Metabolism of acetylcholine by choline esterase present on the post junction membrane.

Substances affecting the neuro muscular transmission are (N M blockers)

a. Competitive inhibitors act on the receptors of post junction membrane. They compete with acetylcholine to bind to the receptors on the motor end plate. When acetylcholine is unable to bind to the receptors, there will not be production of the end plate potential and hence muscle action potential development cannot occur. Unlike acetylcholine, which is metabolized fast, the inhibitors continue to exert action for few hours E.g. *Tubocurarine.*

b. Depolarizing blockers maintain the post junction membrane in depolarized state. When any tissue is in depolarized state it will be refractory to the stimulus. Hence can't produce action potential. *One of the examples of depolarizing blockers is Succinyl CoA that acts much like*

acetylcholine but can't get metabolized fast like acetylcholine.

c. Anticholine esterases inhibit the action of choline esterase and thereby acetylcholine can not get metabolized and continue exert the action for longer duration. *Examples are neostigmine, physostigmine.*

Myasthenia gravis

- Causes weakness or fatigue of muscles because of the inability of the neuro muscular junction to transmit the impulse.
- It is an autoimmune disease.
- The antibodies produced act against the receptors at end plate region and destroy them.
- The decrease in the number of the receptors fails to transmit the impulse.
- If the disease involves the respiratory muscles the person may die.

Patients can be treated with

a. Anti choline esterases like neostigmine to prolong the action of acetylcholine.

b. Thymectomy—removal of thymus to reduce the level of antibodies.

c. Administration of the immuno suppressants to reduce antibody concentration.

EXCITATION CONTRACTION COUPLING (E C COUPLING)

It is a mechanism by which a nerve action potential is converted to muscle action potential and leading to muscle contraction.

Events in excitation contraction coupling and relaxation are Fig. 6.7(a)

- Action potential at the motor nerve ending.
- Release of acetylcholine from the neuron to reach the muscle.

- Development of muscle action potential.
- Spread of the action potential along the T tubules.
- Release of calcium ions from the cisterns.
- Binding of calcium ions to troponin C.
- Formation of cross linkage between actin and myosin due to movement of tropomyosin exposing active sites on actin.
- Sliding of the I band over the A band.
- Z lines come close to each other
- Shortening of muscle.

During relaxation

- Calcium is pumped back into cisterns.
- Release of calcium ions from troponin.
- No interaction between actin and myosin.
- Muscle relaxes.

Muscle contraction summarizing (Fig. 6.8)

a. Z lines move closer.
b. Sarcomere shortens.
c. I band decreases.
d. H band decreases or disappears.
e. A band width remains the same.

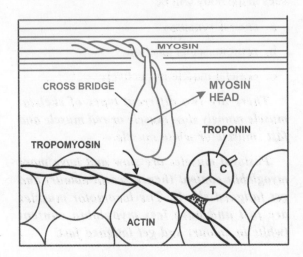
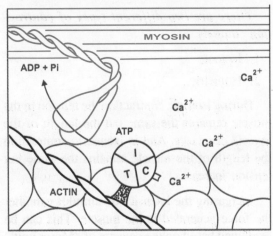

Fig 6.7(a) Process of interaction between actin and myosin during contractions

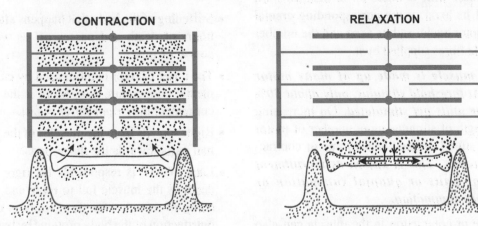

Fig 6.8 Position of Z lines and I band during contraction and relaxation

Properties of skeletal muscle

Excitability

It responds to stimulus. Like in a nerve fibre, even in the muscle, on stimulation there will be development of action potential as the muscle will also be in polarized state at rest. The resting membrane potential in muscle is about –90 mV.

Contractility

Muscle on stimulation with threshold stimulus not only demonstrates the electrical change, there will also be a mechanical change, which is in the form of contraction.

There are two different types of contraction namely

1. Isotonic
2. Isometric.

During isotonic contraction the tension in the muscle remains the same but the length of the muscle decreases. And in isometric contraction the length of the muscle remains the same but tension increases.

Increasing the intensity of stimulus can alter the force generated in the muscle. This can be explained based on the concept of "Motor unit".

A motor unit is made up of anterior horn cell and its axon or the corresponding cranial nerve motor nuclei and its axon and the number of muscle fibres supplied by it.

Any muscle is made up of many motor units. At threshold stimulus, only about 50% of motor units get stimulated. On increasing the strength of stimulus more number of motor unit get stimulated and hence force of contraction increases. *This is known as recruitment of motor units or quantal summation or multifiber summation.*

Force of contraction in the muscle can also be altered based on Starling's law which states that force of contraction is directly proportional to initial length of muscle fibre within physiological limits.

Another way to increase the force of contraction in skeletal muscle will be by bringing about wave summation.

Fatigability

When a tissue is stimulated continuously, in course of time the tissue may fail to respond. This is due to decreased excitability or inability of the tissue to respond. The order of fatigability of the tissues in the body will be

a. central synapses
b. neuromuscular junction
c. skeletal muscle respectively.

There are two different types of skeletal muscle namely slow muscle or red muscle and fast muscle or white muscle.

Postural muscles are slow and have more myoglobin content (hence red in colour) and get fatigued slowly. The locomotor muscles are fast and have less myoglobin content (white in colour) and get fatigued fast.

Rigor mortis

- Stiffening of the body that happens after few hours of death and passes off as well, in course of time.
- The onset of rigor is influenced by environmental temperature also. More is the ambient temperature rigor onset is fast.
- Rigor spreads from the muscles of the proximal parts towards the distal parts.
- Lack of ATP is responsible for rigor. After death as the muscle fail to relax and slackening of muscle after few hours is due to putrifaction of the body proteins by bacterial actions.

SMOOTH MUSCLE

- Are of two types namely visceral and multi unit smooth muscle.
- Smooth muscles in general lack definite cross striations and are involuntary in function.
- The smooth muscle activity is nerve regulated unlike the skeletal muscle which is nerve operated.
  Hence the skeletal muscle undergoes paralysis when motor neuron supplying the muscle is damaged.

Visceral or single unit or unitary smooth muscle is found in gastro intestinal tract, urinary bladder, uterus etc. They possess spontaneous electrical activity and cell-to-cell conduction of the impulse is possible. The sympathetic and parasympathetic nerve supplying them can alter the rate of activity.

Multiunit smooth muscle is found in iris, ciliaris muscle, erector pilorum etc. In this type of muscle there is no cell-to-cell conduction of impulse and no spontaneous activity. Sympathetic and parasympathetic nerves supply them and stimulation of the nerves can alter the activity.

Smooth muscles in general have the property of excitability, conductivity, contractility etc. *One of the important properties of visceral smooth muscle is plasticity.* Because of this, almost the same pressure is maintained despite change in the length of muscle fibres.

7

Respiratory System

- Introduction
- Lungs and structure of respiratory tract
- Pressure changes during respiration
- Spirogram
- Exchange of gases at lungs
- Oxygen transport
- Carbon dioxide transport
- Regulation of respiration
- Hypoxia
- Acclimatization
- Decompression sickness and periodic breathing

INTRODUCTION

The respiratory system is concerned with delivery of oxygen from the atmosphere to tissues and excretion of carbon dioxide from the tissues to atmosphere. Oxygen diffuses into blood at the level of lungs and at the same time carbon dioxide is evolved out of blood into lungs.

Exchange of gases at the level of lungs is known as external respiration.

At the level of tissues, *the reversal occurs. Oxygen is diffused into tissues from blood and at the same time carbon dioxide is diffused into blood from the tissues. This is known as internal respiration.*

Respiratory tract

Parts of respiratory system starting from the nasal apertures, extends through pharynx, larynx, trachea, bronchi, bronchioles and into alveoli. *Alveolus is the structural and functional unit of respiratory system*. The part extending from the nasal apertures upto bronchioles (terminal bronchioles) forms the respiratory tract & is also known as conducting zone. This region is known as anatomical dead space.

The concept of dead space is part of respiratory system in which inspite of air being present it doesn't take part in exchange of

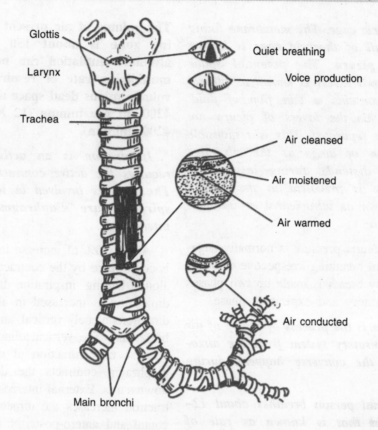

Fig 7.1 Diagram of tracheobronchial tree

gases. The normal anatomical dead space air is about 150 ml (DSA).

Functions of upper respiratory tract
(Fig. 7.1)

1. Warming up of air, as the temperature of air reaching the alveoli should be brought to body temperature, for better diffusion of gas.

2. The epithelial cells lining the respiratory tract add on water molecules to the air getting into the alveoli. This is known as humidifying of air.

3. Filtration of air is essential before the air reaches alveoli. Partial filtration of dust particles will be taking place due to the presence of the ciliated cells on which a layer of mucus is present.

All the aforesaid aspects in general are known as air conditioning. In addition to this the passage of air through the larynx is responsible for production of sound.

LUNGS

Human beings have a pair of lungs, which are present in thoracic cavity. A membrane known as visceral pleura covers the lungs. This layer gets reflected and continues to form a membrane covering on the inner wall of thoracic cage. The membrane lining the inner wall of thoracic cage is known as parietal pleura. The potential space between the two layers is known as pleural space that contains a thin film of fluid. Because of this the layers of pleura are unable to get separated. This is responsible for distension of lungs as the rib cage expands or distends during inspiration. Pressure that is prevalent in the pleural space is known as intrapleural or intrathoracic pressure.

The intrapleural pressure is normally negative in normal breathing irrespective of phase of breath. Any breath is made up two phases namely inspiratory and expiratory phase.

Inspiration is the process of entry of air into the respiratory system from the atmosphere and the converse happens during expiration.

Any normal person breathes about 12–15 times/min that is known as rate of respiration. The volume of air that is taken in or given out of respiratory system during a normal quiet breathing is known as tidal volume. The normal tidal volume is about 500 ml.

Pulmonary ventilation *is defined as the volume of air entering or leaving the respiratory system per minute. So it is the product of rate of respiration (RR) multiplied by tidal volume (TV), which is about 6000 ml normally (12 × 500 = 6000 ml/min).*

Alveolar ventilation **is defined as the volume of air taking part in the exchange of gases at the level of alveoli per minute. As stated already the alveolar area region is where the exchange of gas occurs but the air present in the conducting zone doesn't take part in exchange of gases.**

The volume of air present in the conducting zone is about 150 ml (DSA). So alveolar ventilation can be calculated by multiplying rate of respiration and tidal volume minus dead space air and is about 4200 ml per minute (12 × 500 − 150 = 4200 ml/min).

Inspiration is an active process that requires the active contraction of muscles. The muscles involved in normal quiet inspiration are diaphragm and external intercostals.

About 70% of increase in thoracic volume is contributed by the contraction of diaphragm alone. During inspiration the thoracic cage dimension is increased in all the 3 different directions namely vertical, antero-posterior and horizontal. The vertical dimension increase is because of contraction of diaphragm. When diaphragm contracts the diaphragm moves downwards. External intercostals muscles contraction increases the dimension in the horizontal and antero-posterior directions.

The normal quiet expiration is a passive process, which is due to the elastic recoiling of the alveoli. When the distended alveoli of inspiratory phase get recoiled during expiration adequate pressure is built up in the alveoli to force out the air from lungs into atmosphere during quiet respiration.

Phrenic nerve (root value C_{3-5}) supplies the diaphragm and intercostal nerves (root value $T_1—T_{11}$) supply the intercostal muscles. **In addition to these muscles, some of the other muscles are also involved in deep inspiration or expiration. They are called accessory muscles of inspiration or expiration.** *The accessory muscles of inspirations are sternocleidomastoid, serratus anterior etc and that of expiration are rectus abdominus, internal oblique, internal intercostal.*

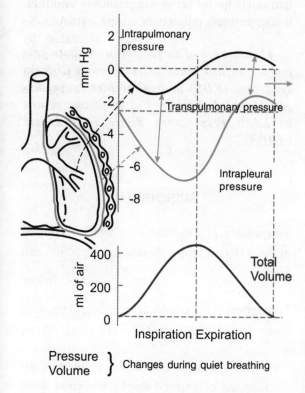

Fig 7.2 Diagram of intrapleural and intraalveolar pressures with tidal volume.

PRESSURE CHANGES DURING RESPIRATION

Intrapleural pressure or intrathoracic pressure (Fig. 7.2) is the pressure recorded in the pleural space. *It is always subatmospheric whether during inspiration or expiration. At the beginning of inspiration it is –3 mm Hg and at the end of inspiration it becomes – 6 mm Hg and at the end of expiration comes back to – 3 mm Hg. It is only when there is expiration against closed glottis the intrapleural pressure can become positive. In deep inspiration it can become more negative.*

The negative intrapleural pressure

1. Facilitates continuous venous drainage to heart by maintaining the patency of veins in the thoracic region.

2. Helps for movement of air across the bronchioles both during inspiration and expiration by maintaining the patency of the lumen.

3. Helps to maintain continuous lymph drainage through the thoracic duct.

4. Reduces collapsing tendency of the alveoli.

Intraalveolar pressure or intrapulmonary pressure (Fig. 7.2) is the pressure recorded from the alveoli. *Unlike the intrapleural pressure, which is always negative, the intraalveolar pressure becomes negative during inspiration and positive during expiration. This facilitates the movement of air into or out of alveoli. The alveoli are connected to atmosphere through the respiratory tract. The movement of air is always along the pressure gradient.* As the atmospheric pressure usually can't be altered easily, a change in the intraalveolar pressure has to be brought about to achieve the necessary gradient for the movement of air in any specific direction.

The intraalveolar pressure become minus 1 mm Hg by mid inspiration from the 0 mm Hg at the beginning of inspiration. During the 2nd half of inspiratory phase it returns to 0 mm Hg. During early expiratory phase it becomes plus 1 mm Hg and at the end of expiration it returns to 0 mm Hg.

The difference between the intrapleural and intraalveolar pressure is known as transpulmonary pressure. Because the lungs have the ability to get distended, a change in the volume of lung occurs when the lung get inflated or deflated. The change in the volume of lung per unit change in transpulmonary pressure is known as compliance of lung. It is about 200 ml per cm H_2O (Fig. 7.3). *The compliance of lung is affected in pulmonary edema, fibrosis of lungs, emphysema, age. Compliance can be calculated with the help of the following formula*

$$\text{(Compliance) } C = \frac{\text{delta V (volume)}}{\text{delta P (pressure)}}$$

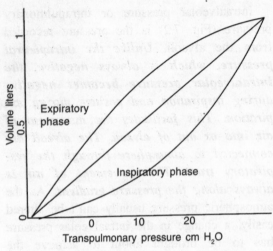

Fig 7.3 Graph indicating lung compliance

Surfactant is the lipid protein complex (di palmitoyl phosphotidyl choline) secreted by type II alveolar epithelial cells (pneumocytes). It starts getting secreted in the last trimester (7th month) of pregnancy. **It forms an inter phase between the fluid present in the alveoli and the air in the alveoli. And hence it decreases the surface tension in the lungs.**

Secretion of surfactant is affected by the action of the hormone thyroxine and maturation of the secreted surfactant is influenced by the hormone cortisol. About 2/3 rd of collapsing tendency of the alveoli is prevented by the surfac-

tant and helps for better compliance in the lungs. It also prevents pulmonary edema formation.

The absence of surfactant in newborn premature infant leads to respiratory distress syndrome (RDS) or hyaline membrane disease. In adult deficiency of surfactant results in adult respiratory distress syndrome (ARDS).

SPIROGRAM

Spirometry is a technique by which recording of the different lung volumes and capacities can be done.

Spirogram is the graphical recording of the lung volumes and capacities (Fig. 7.4).

- **Tidal volume (TV)** is the volume of air inspired or expired during a normal quiet respiration and it is about 500 ml.

- **Inspiratory reserve volume (IRV)** is the volume of air inspired forcibly after a tidal inspiration — 3000 ml.

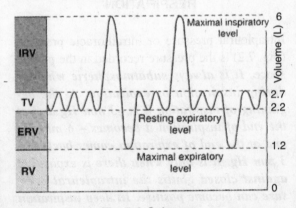

Fig 7.4 Spirogram

- **Expiratory reserve volume (ERV)** is the volume of air expired forcibly after tidal expiration — 1100 ml.

- **Residual volume (RV)** is the volume of air remaining in the lungs even after a forced expiration — 1200 ml.

A capacity is sum of two or more different lung volumes.

- **Functional residual capacity (FRC)** is the volume of air remaining in the lungs after a normal expiration (RV + ERV) and is about 2300 ml. This air is responsible for continuous exchange of gases irrespective of phase of respiration.

- **Total lung capacity** is the maximum volume of air present in the lungs after a forced inspiration. It is sum of IRV, TV, ERV and RV, which is around 6000 ml.

- **Vital capacity (VC)** is the volume of air expired forcibly after a maximal inspiration. It includes TV, ERV and IRV. Normally it is about 4600 ml.

In relation to body surface area vital capacity is about 2.8 L/m sq in males and 2.3 L/m sq in females.

Vital capacity determination forms one of the important lung function tests. It is normal in obstructive type of lung diseases and decreased in restrictive type of lung diseases.

Vital capacity is also dependent on the age, sex and build of the individual.

Vital capacity decreases in fibrosis of lungs, paralysis of respiratory muscles.

Timed vital capacity (Fig. 7.5) is the percentage volume of vital capacity expired at the end of successive seconds. Usually it is denoted as FEV_1, FEV_2 and FEV_3 wherein FEV refers to the forced expiratory volume and the number suffixed refers to the end of a particular second. To calculate timed vital capacity at the end of one second the following formula can be applied

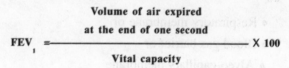

$$FEV_1 = \frac{\text{Volume of air expired at the end of one second}}{\text{Vital capacity}} \times 100$$

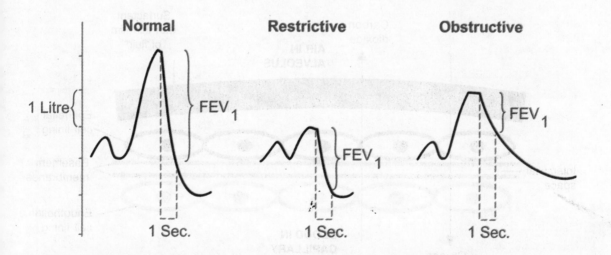

Fig 7.5 Diagram indicating the variations in VC and TVC in certain respiratory diseases

Normal value:

FEV_1 is 75–80%

FEV_2 is 85–90%

FEV_3 is about 97%

Timed vital capacity decreases in obstructive type of lung diseases (bronchial asthma) even though vital capacity remains normal. Vital capacity is decreased in restrictive type of lung diseases but the timed vital capacity remains normal.

EXCHANGE OF GAS AT LUNGS

The gases diffuse across the respiratory membrane in lungs. Oxygen diffuses into blood from lungs and carbon dioxide diffuses out of blood into the lungs. The membrane across which the gaseous exchange occurs is known as

- Respiratory membrane or
- Blood gas barrier or
- Alveo-capillary membrane

The membrane is made up of (Fig. 7.6)

- Surfactant with thin film of fluid
- Alveolar epithelial cell layer
- Basement membrane of alveolar epithelium
- Interstitium of lungs
- Basement membrane of pulmonary capillary.
- Capillary endothelium

Even though it is made up so many layers the thickness of the membrane is about 0.5 microns.

Diffusion

Volume of gas diffusing across the membrane is directly proportional to (based on Fick's law of diffusion)

- Partial pressure gradient for the gas
- Surface area available for diffusion
- Solubility of the gas

And inversely related to

- Thickness of the membrane
- Square root of molecular weight of gas.

Among the aforesaid factors, the solubility and

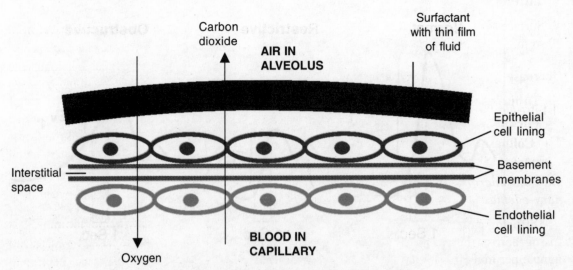

Fig 7.6 Diagram of respiratory membrane

square root of molecular weight of gases are constant. Carbon dioxide is 24 times more soluble than oxygen but in relation to square root of molecular weight, oxygen has a better diffusing capability. When both the factors are considered the diffusing capability is 20:1 for carbon dioxide and oxygen respectively.

Hence a variation in pressure gradient or surface area availability or thickness of the membrane will alter the volume of gas getting diffused.

Accordingly the partial pressure gradient available for oxygen diffusion in normal conditions at sea level is about 64 mm Hg and for carbon dioxide it is about 6 mm Hg. Eventhough the pressure gradient available for carbon dioxide diffusion is only about $1/10^{th}$ of oxygen, still it is able to diffuse easily because carbon dioxide diffusing ability is about 20 times more when compared to oxygen.

Pressure gradient gets affected in conditions like

- **Hypoventilation of alveoli (bronchial asthma)**
- **Hyperventilation of alveoli (at high altitudes)**

Surface area availability is normally around 70 sq m.

Decrease in surface area occurs in

- **Tuberculosis**
- **Pneumonia**
- **Collpase of lung lobes**

Thickness of the respiratory membrane *is only 0.5 microns. It is increased in pulmonary edema.*

Diffusing capacity is the volume of gas diffusing across the respiratory membrane per minute per mm Hg pressure gradient. For oxygen it is about *21 ml/ mm Hg/ minute.*

OXYGEN TRANSPORT

- Volume present in 100 ml of blood
- Partial pressure at different regions
- Forms of transport
- Importance of dissolved form
- In combination with hemoglobin
- Oxygen hemoglobin dissociation curve and factors influencing

In 100 ml of blood the volume of oxygen present in

- **Arterial blood is about 20 ml**
- **Venous blood is about 15 ml (mixed venous blood in right ventricle/ pulmonary artery)**

Partial pressure at different regions is

- Arterial blood 95 mm Hg.
- Tissues < 40 mm Hg.
- Venous blood 40 mm Hg (mixed venous blood in right ventricle/pulmonary artery)
- Alveoli 104 mm Hg at sea level.

So when pulmonary arterial blood, which contains mixed venous blood, flows through the lungs, there will be a pressure gradient of about 64 mm Hg for the diffusion of oxygen into blood from the alveoli. In about $1/3^{rd}$ the distance of the pulmonary capillary and time available in lungs, the pressure equilibration is brought about between alveolar air and blood. This acts as safety factor for better oxygenation in muscular exercise wherein the rate of flow of blood through the pulmonary circulation will be very fast.

Forms of transport are

- **Dissolved form**
- **In combination with hemoglobin.**

In the dissolved form it is about 0.3 ml/100 ml of blood in the arterial blood and 0.1 ml/ 100 ml of blood in the venous blood. *But still this particular form of transport is very essential as this form of gas alone can exerts partial pressure that is necessary for diffusion of any gas. Oxygen gets dissolved in water available both in plasma and red blood cells.*

Oxygen is transported by hemoglobin as well. *Volume of oxygen transported by hemoglobin in the arterial blood is about 19.5 ml/ 100 ml and in venous blood it is about 14.5 ml/ 100 ml.*

$$Hb + O_2 \rightleftarrows HbO_2$$

So the percentage saturation of hemoglobin is about

- 97% in arterial blood (oxygenated blood)
- 70% in the venous blood. (Deoxygenated blood)

Percentage saturation of hemoglobin is ratio between volume of oxygen carried by 1 gm of hemoglobin to the maximum oxygen carrying capacity of hemoglobin times hundred.

$$\% \text{ Saturation of Hb} = \frac{\text{Volume of } O_2 \text{ carried by 1 gm Hb}}{\text{Maximum } O_2 \text{ carrying ability of 1 gm Hb}} \times 100$$

One gram of hemoglobin can carry about 1.34 ml of oxygen on full saturation.

Even though about 20 ml of oxygen is available in arterial blood for utilization by the tissues, the tissues normally use only 5 ml of oxygen when 100 ml of blood flows through them. In other words only a part of oxygen available to them gets utilized. This is known as utilization coefficient. The ratio between the volume of oxygen used to the volume of oxygen available for utilization by the tissues is known as utilization coefficient. The utilization coefficient of oxygen is normally about 25%. *In severe muscular*

exercise it can go upto about 75%.

Oxygen binds to the heme part of hemoglobin. The reaction is a physical one. The reaction will be oxygenation and not oxidation, as the ferrous form of iron in hemoglobin does not get oxidsed to ferric form. Each molecule of hemoglobin with 4 atoms of iron can carry 4 molecules of oxygen. The reactions occur in step wise and it is known as heme-heme interaction. This type of binding of oxygen facilitates the rate of binding of oxygen to hemoglobin.

Oxygen dissociation curve (Fig. 7.7)

It is the graphical representation of % saturation of hemoglobin in relation to partial pressure of oxygen.

Factors affecting dissociation are

- **Partial pressure of carbon dioxide**
- **H^+ in blood (pH)**
- **Temperature**
- **Conc. of 2-3 DPG**

Increase of all of the above factors shift

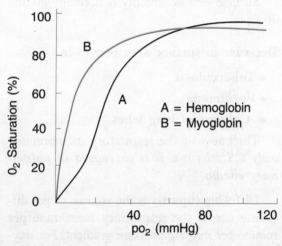

Fig 7.7 Graph showing oxygen dissociation curve

the dissociation curve to right. Increase in pCO_2 or decrease in pH, which shifts the curve to right, is known as Bohr's effect. The dissociation curve configuration varies for fetal hemoglobin and myoglobin.

P_{50} is the partial pressure of oxygen at which hemoglobin is saturated to 50%. At sea level it is about 28 mm Hg.

CARBON DIOXIDE TRANSPORT

- Content
- Partial pressure at different regions
- Forms of transport
- Importance of dissolved form
- In combination with hemoglobin
- Carbon dioxide dissociation curve and factors influencing the same.

Content

In arterial blood it is about 48 ml / 100 ml of blood and in the venous blood (mixed) is about 52 ml/ 100 ml.

Partial pressure at different regions

- Arterial blood is 40 mm Hg.
- In tissues is about 46 mm Hg.
- In venous blood it is 46 mm Hg. (mixed venous blood)
- In alveoli around 40 mm Hg.

Forms of transport

- Dissolved form
- As bicarbonate
- As carbamino compound

Dissolved form

In arterial blood it is about 2.5 ml and in venous blood it is about 2.8 ml per 100 ml of blood. It is this form of gas that exerts partial pressure. It gets dissolved in water available in plasma and red blood cells.

Carbon dioxide is transported as bicarbonate both in red blood cells and plasma. But the formation of bicarbonate occurs only in erythrocytes because of the presence of the enzyme carbonic anhydrase. Bicarbonate thus formed inside the red blood cells, diffuses into the plasma along the concentration gradient.

At the tissue level when oxygen gets diffused from blood, simultaneously carbon dioxide gets diffused from the tissues into blood. This carbon dioxide apart from getting dissolved in water present in the plasma, some amount also gets diffused into the red blood cells. In the erythrocytes also some amount is transported in the dissolved form. However the presence of carbonic anhydrase enzyme in red blood cell facilitates the reaction between carbon dioxide and water and there will be formation of carbonic acid. This acid is an unstable acid. Immediately it dissociates to form bicarbonate and hydrogen ion. Hemoglobin that has liberated oxygen buffers the hydrogen ion that is formed during the reaction between carbon dioxide and water. When hemoglobin reacts with hydrogen ion, the hemoglobin now is called reduced hemoglobin. The reduced hemoglobin reacts with carbon di oxide to form carbamino hemoglobin, which is also one of the forms of carbon dioxide transport. Unlike oxygen that binds to the heme part, carbon dioxide is attached to the globin part of hemoglobin (Fig.7.8).

Bicarbonate thus formed inside the red blood cell diffuses into plasma along the concentration gradient. Electrical activity of both red blood cells and plasma gets affected since bicarbonate is a charged ion. In order to maintain an electrical neutrality, when bicarbonate diffuse out of cells, chloride ion

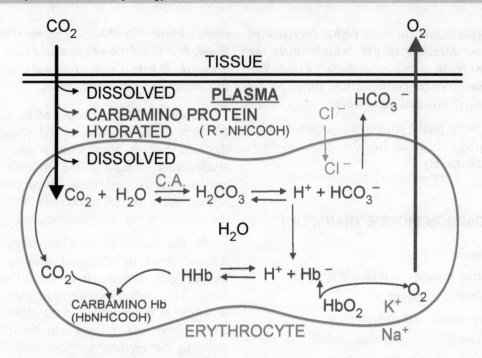

Fig 7.8 Diagram showing the reaction of carbon dioxide in blood at tissue level

diffuses into red blood cells from the plasma. This is known as **chloride shift or Hamburger's** phenomenon. This will be followed by diffusion of water into the red blood cells to maintain the tonicity.

The whole set of reactions get reversed at the level of lungs during the process of diffusion of gas and thereby leads to the oxygenation of blood.

Carbon dioxide dissociation curve (Fig. 7.9)

Graphical relation between partial pressure of carbon dioxide and volume of carbon dioxide in 100 ml of blood.

Shift of the curve to right is due to increase in the partial pressure of oxygen and is known as Haldane's effect. Haldane's effect will help both the uptake (at tissue level) as well as giving out of carbon dioxide (at lungs).

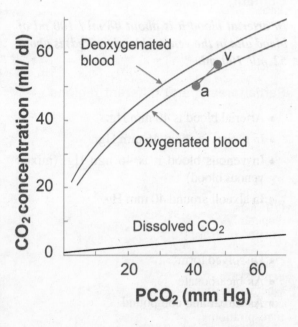

Fig 7.9 Carbon dioxide dissociation curve

REGULATION OF RESPIRATION

Is entirely due to neural mechanism. But the chemical and non-chemical influences can act on the neural mechanism to alter the respiration (Fig. 7.10). *There should be a constant monitoring of respiration in order to maintain the partial pressure and content of various gases in our body to meet the oxygen demand by the tissues and to remove carbon dioxide which is a metabolic waste product.*

Neural mechanism

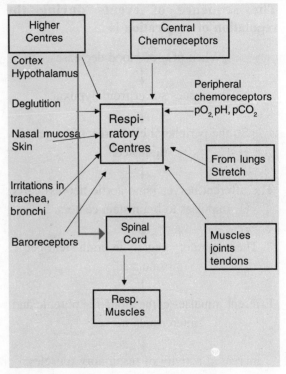

Fig 7.10 Various influences acting on the respiratory centres

Centres are present in brain stem. The brain stem centers are required for rhythmic respiration whether during asleep or awake. The cerebral cortical center is required for voluntary alterations in respiration.

Brain stem centers are present in the reticular formation of pons and medulla oblongata.

In the pons the centers present are

- Pneumotaxic • Apneustic.

In medulla oblongata the centers present are

- Inspiratory (dorso medial group of neurons)
- Expiratory (ventro lateral group of neurons)

There is a lot of interconnection between the various centers. The interplay of the different centers is essential for a proper regulation of respiration. The medullary centers are termed as primary/basic centers, whereas the pontine centers are called regulatory centers. The pontine centers act through the medullary centers for smooth rhythmic respiration to be brought about.

From the medullary centers the impulses are sent to spinal cord through the reticulospinal pathway, which ends on the anterior horn cells in spinal cord. Both the phrenic and intercostal nerve take origin from spinal cord and influence the activity of diaphragm and intercostals muscles respectively which are the muscles of normal quiet respiration.

So if there is a transverse section of spinal cord at the level of

- C_2 segment person dies of respiratory paralysis.
- C_6 person may survive because the diaphragmatic respiration continues.

The apneustic center controls the activity of inspiratory center. The apneustic center activity in turn is controlled by the impulses coming from the pneumotaxic center and through the vagus nerve from the stretch receptors of lungs. When the influence by the vagus and pneumotaxic center over the apneustic center is lost, there will be prolonged inspiration and a sudden expiration. This type of breathing is known as apneustic breathing.

Sequence of events during normal regulation of respiration by neural mechanism

- Impulse from the apneustic center stimulates the inspiratory center.
- Stimulation of inspiratory center leads to
    a. Impulses being sent to spinal cord for stimulation of phrenic and intercostals nerves
    b. Reciprocal inhibition of expiratory center
    c. Excitatory impulses sent to pneumotaxic center through multisynaptic pathway.
- When inspiration is going on, there will be gradual inhibition of the apneustic center by the impulses coming from the pneumotaxic center and also from the vagal fibres of the distended lungs.
- This leads to no excitatory inputs to inspiratory center. Hence the activity of this center stops and leads to no inhibition of the expiratory center by inspiratory center.
- Now loss of inhibitory influence from inspiratory center leads to expiratory center becoming active.
- The muscles of inspiration start relaxing due to no impulses along the phrenic and intercostals nerves. The relaxation of the muscles is more than enough to bring about a normal quiet expiration.

Chemical regulation of respiration

This is brought about by the chemoreceptors. They are called

- Peripheral
- Central chemoreceptors.

The peripheral chemoreceptors are present in

a. Carotid bodies which are present at the branching of common carotid artery.

b. Aortic bodies that are present in arch of aorta.

The afferent impulses from the carotid bodies will be carried by sinus nerve branch of glassopharyngeal nerve and from the aortic bodies by aortic nerve branch of vagus nerve.

The peripheral chemoreceptors respond to

- **Decrease in pO_2**
- **Increase in H^+**
- **Increase of pCO_2 of blood.**

The sequence of events during the regulation of respiration is

When pO_2 of blood decreases

↓

The tissues suffer from hypoxia.

↓

So the peripheral chemoreceptors get stimulated.

↓

The afferent nerves (sino aortic nerves) carry impulses to brain stem centers.

↓

The respiratory centers in brain stem get stimulated.

↓

Efferent impulses come along the phrenic and intercostals nerves.

↓

Increased activity of respiratory muscles.

↓

Increase in the rate and depth of respiration.

↓

Increased diffusion of gases across the respiratory membrane.

↓

Increase partial pressure of oxygen in the blood, which ensures more oxygen delivery to the tissues.

Central chemoreceptors

They are present in the brain stem near the respiratory centers. They are more sensitive to hydrogen ions, but the hydrogen ion of blood can't stimulate them because the blood brain barrier is impermeable for the hydrogen ion to diffuse through. Hence the increase in partial pressure of carbon dioxide forms the stimulus.

Sequence of events

Increase pCO_2 in blood.

↓

Carbon dioxide diffuses across the blood brain barrier into the neural tissue.

↓

Carbon dioxide reacts with water to form carbonic acid.

↓

This acid dissociates into hydrogen and bicarbonate ions.

↓

Hydrogen ion stimulates central chemoreceptors.

↓

They in turn stimulate respiratory centers.

↓

This increases the activity of respiratory muscles due to increased impulses through the motor nerves.

↓

There will be increase in the respiratory activity.

↓

Increased diffusion of gases across the respiratory membrane and elimination of more carbon dioxide from the body.

↓

Decreases pCO_2.

Non-chemical influences on respiratory centers pertain to impulses coming from

- Irritant receptors stimulation in lungs while coughing.
- Receptors of muscles and joints.
- Irritation of nasal mucosa (sneezing)
- Mechanoreceptors in pharynx (deglutition).

Depending on the location of the receptors influencing the respiratory centers, there will be appropriate alterations in the respiration.

Cyanosis

a. Cyanosis is the bluish discoloration of skin and mucus membrane.

b. It occurs due to an increase in the concentration of reduced hemoglobin in capillary blood.

c. The concentration of reduced hemoglobin when exceeds 5 g%, there will be cyanosis.

d. Cyanosis can be central or peripheral.

e. Usually it is obvious in lips, nail beds.

f. Cyanosis occurs in hypoxic hypoxia and stagnant hypoxia.

g. It can occur when there is problem with lungs or heart as disease of either organs decreases the diffusion of oxygen across the lungs.

HYPOXIA

When there is deficient oxygen supply to the tissues it is called hypoxia.

Depending on the problem, there are 4 types of hypoxias. They are

- Hypoxic hypoxia
- Anemic hypoxia
- Stagnant hypoxia
- Histotoxic hypoxia

Hypoxic hypoxia occurs when there is, decrease in alveolar ventilation (asthma), pulmonary edema, heart diseases, decrease of pressure in atomosphere at high altitudes.

Some of the features are

- $\Downarrow$ pO_2 in arterial blood.
- % Saturation of hemoglobin $\Downarrow$
- Arterial oxygen content decreased
- Oxygen carrying capacity of hemoglobin is normal.
- $\Uparrow$ In the concentration of reduced hemoglobin in capillary blood.
- Cyanosis occurs

Anemic hypoxia occurs due to quantitative decrease in hemoglobin (anemias) or qualitative defect in hemoglobin (carbon monoxide poisoning).

Some of the features are

- Normal pO_2 in arterial blood
- % Saturation of hemoglobin normal
- Arterial oxygen content decreased
- Oxygen carrying capacity of blood decreased
- Concentration of reduced hemoglobin normal

Stagnant hypoxia occurs in decreased rate of blood flow as seen in heart failures, cardio vascular shocks, obstruction in the blood vessels.

Some of the features are

- Normal pO_2 in arterial blood
- % Saturation of hemoglobin normal
- Oxygen content normal in arterial blood
- Oxygen carrying capacity of hemoglobin normal
- Concentration of reduced hemoglobin increases in capillary blood
- Cyanosis occurs.

Histotoxic hypoxia occurs in poisoning of tissues. The cytochrome oxidase and mitochondrial activity is affected in this condition. This occurs in cyanide poisoning.

Some of the features are

- Normal pO_2 in arterial blood
- % Saturation of hemoglobin normal
- Arterial oxygen content normal
- Oxygen carrying capacity of hemoglobin normal
- Concentration of reduced hemoglobin is less

Apnoea is temporary cessation of breathing. The different types are

- Deglutition apnoea (during deglutition)
- Voluntary apnoea when breath is held voluntarily.
- Vagal apnoea
- Adrenaline apnoea
- Hyperventilation apnoea.

ACCLIMATIZATION

Acclimatization can be defined as the physiological changes that are brought about to adjust for an altered atmosphere when exposed for prolonged duration.

Some of the physiological changes occur when the body is exposed to high altitudes are

- Increase of rate and depth of respiration.
- Increase in myoglobin content.
- Increase of cytochrome oxidase enzyme activity.
- Increase in mitochondria.
- Increased number of capillaries through which blood flows.
- Increase of red blood cell count.
- Increase of cardiac output.

All the above changes help the person to sustain life easily even at a higher altitude.

DECOMPRESSION SICKNESS/CAISSON'S DISEASE/DYSBARISM

Occurs when people exposed to high barometric pressure suddenly get exposed to low atmospheric pressure. Usually seen in divers. At high pressures more gas will have gone into the dissolved state in all the tissues of body including blood. So when the atomospheric pressure decreases, these gases will get bubbled out. Because of the bubbling of gases either in tissues or in the blood stream, it can lead to certain problems. Some of the features of the condition are

- Compression in chest
- Pain in the joints
- Pain at the back
- Itching
- At times there can be damage to brain tissue as well, which may lead to paresis.

Treatment

Promote recompression in a chamber and perform slow decompression.

Asphyxia

Is a condition in which there will be hypoxia (decrease in pO_2) and hypercapnia (increase in pCO_2) in the body occurring simultaneously. Asphyxia occurs in strangulation, obstruction to the air passage.

Dyspnoea means difficulty to breathe. Classical example where dysnoea seen is in bronchial asthma.

Periodic breathing is where the breaths are interposed with some amount of apnoea. The different types of periodic breathing are (Fig. 7.11)

- Cheyne-Stokes
- Biot's
- Kussmaul.

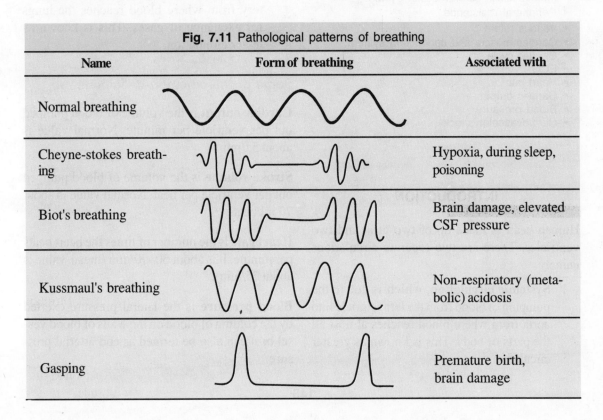

Fig. 7.11 Pathological patterns of breathing

Name	Form of breathing	Associated with
Normal breathing		
Cheyne-stokes breathing		Hypoxia, during sleep, poisoning
Biot's breathing		Brain damage, elevated CSF pressure
Kussmaul's breathing		Non-respiratory (metabolic) acidosis
Gasping		Premature birth, brain damage

8

Cardiovascular System

- Introduction
- Innervation to cardiovascular system
- Peripheral resistence
- Venous return
- Cardiac muscle and conducting system
- Cardiac cycle
- ECG
- Heart rate
- Cardiac output
- Blood pressure
- Cardiovascular shock

INTRODUCTION

Human heart is made up of two atria and two ventricles. There are two separate circulations namely

1. **Systemic circulation, which** is due to the pumping of blood from the left ventricle into aorta from where blood reaches almost all the parts of body. This is known as greater circulation.

2. **Pulmonary circulation** is pumping of blood from the right ventricle into pulmonary artery from where blood reaches the lungs for exchange of gases. This is known as lesser circulation.

Some of the common definitions are

Cardiac output is the volume of blood pumped out per ventricle per minute. Normal value is about 5 l/min.

Stroke volume is the volume of blood pumped out per ventricle per beat. Normal value is about 70 ml/beat.

Heart rate is the number of times the heart beats per minute. It is about 60–90/min (mean value is about 75/min).

Blood pressure is the lateral pressure exerted by the column of blood on the walls of blood vessel or it can also be termed as end arterial pressure.

Peripheral resistance is the resistance offered by the vessel wall on the flowing column of blood.

Sympathetic tone/arteriolar tone is the constant excitatory influence by the sympathetic fibres on smooth muscle in the wall of the arterioles.

Venomotor tone is the constant excitatory influence by the sympathetic fibres on smooth muscle on the wall of the veins.

Autorhythmicity is the ability of the tissue to generate its own impulse at regular intervals.

Pace maker is the region that sets the pace at which the heart has to beat in unit time. Normally SA node (sino atrial node) acts as the pacemaker in human heart.

Vagal tone is the constant inhibitory influence exerted by vagus nerve on heart.

ECG (electrocardiogram) is the graphical recording of the summated electrical activity from the heart.

Cardiac cycle is the sequential changes brought about during the heartbeat.

Systole is the contractile state of atrium/ventricle during a cardiac cycle.

Diastole is the relaxation state of atrium/ventricle during a cardiac cycle.

Innervation of cardio vascular system

The nerves belonging to autonomic nervous system supply structures of cardio vascular system. The nerves included under autonomic nervous system are

- Sympathetic
- Parasympathetic.

Nerve supply to heart

Parasympathetic is by vagus nerve which takes origin from the dorsal motor nucleus present in the floor of the 4th ventricle.

Sympathetic nerves take origin from the lateral horn cells of T_1–T_5 segments in spinal cord.

Nerve supply to the smooth muscle of blood vessels is predominantly the sympathetic nerves. They take origin from the lateral horn cells of T_1–L_2 segments in spinal cord.

Details of vascular tree

Aorta is known as damping vessel, which has more amount of elastic tissue in the walls. In this vessel, the intermittent ejection of blood from the ventricle into the arterial vessels (during ventricular systole) is converted into a continuous flow in blood vessels (throughout the cardiac cycle). Thereby it acts as a secondary pump, the primary pump being the left ventricle.

Arterioles are known as resistance vessels. Lot of smooth muscle is present in the walls of these blood vessels. The contractility of the smooth muscle can alter the lumen diameter of the blood vessels. Alteration in the lumen diameter affects the peripheral resistance. The smooth muscle contractility is constantly under the influence of sympathetic nerves because of arteriolar tone. Due to the peripheral resistance, the diastolic blood pressure is maintained.

Capillaries are known as exchange vessels. They are thin walled with a layer of endothelial cells. The exchange of substances between blood and tissue takes place only at the level of capillaries.

Veins are known as capacitance vessels. In the whole of vascular tree, the lumen diameter is maximum at this region and vessel wall is very thin. Any alteration in the circulating volume of blood can be brought about by appropriate changes in lumen diameter without affecting the pressure considerably. The wall contains some amount of smooth muscle whose activity is also under the control sympathetic nerves.

PERIPHERAL RESISTANCE

Peripheral resistance is the resistance offered by the wall of the blood vessel on blood flowing through. *It is maximum at the arteriolar region.* Hence arterioles are known as seat of maximum peripheral resistance. *The maintenance of peripheral resistance is essential as peripheral resistance affects the diastolic blood pressure. Peripheral resistance and diastolic blood pressure have direct relationship. Peripheral resistance is also affected by viscosity of blood.*

The arteriolar smooth muscle contractility is under the influence of

- Impulses coming through the sympathetic nerves increase the contractility.
- Certain chemical substances present in circulation, which can either enhance or decrease the contractility.
- Certain tissue metabolites as well can alter the contractile state.

Sympathetic vasoconstrictor tone (Fig. 8.1)

Of all the above factors the role of sympathetic

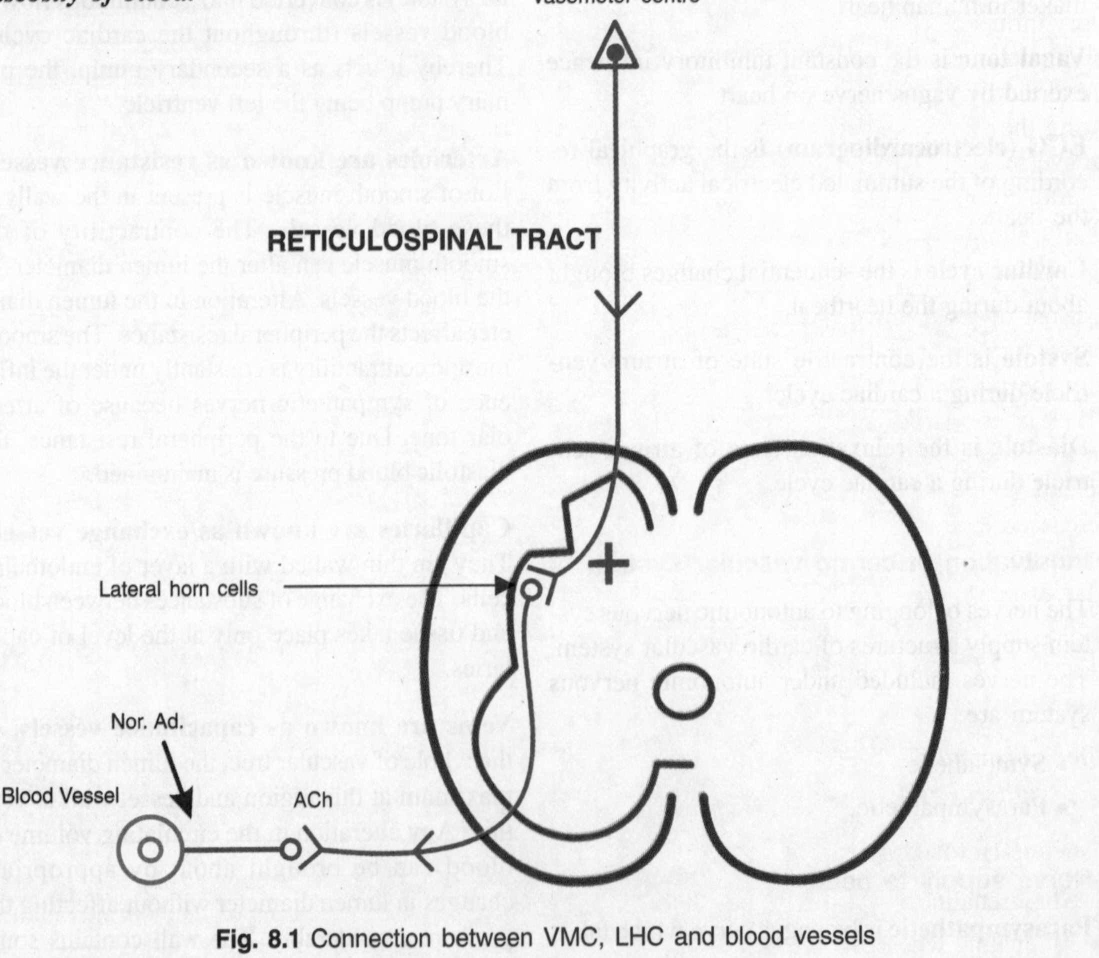

Fig. 8.1 Connection between VMC, LHC and blood vessels

nerves on vascular smooth muscle is very important. The nerve supply to the vascular smooth muscle comes from the lateral horn cells of T_1–L_2 segments of spinal cord. There will be constant excitatory influence by the sympathetic efferent fibres on the smooth muscle of arterioles. This is known as sympathetic tone or arteriolar tone.

The impulses from a center present in the reticular formation of brain stem in turn influence the activity of the sympathetic nerves of spinal cord. The center is known as vasomotor center (VMC). Vasomotor center keeps sending impulses to the lateral horn cells of spinal cord through reticulospinal tract. Hence the sympathetic nerves constantly exert a stimulatory influence on the arteriolar smooth muscle and maintain peripheral resistance. When the lateral horn cells activity is depressed (seen during the stage of spinal shock after complete transverse section of spinal cord) there will be general fall of blood pressure. This is mainly due to the loss of sympathetic influence on arteriolar smooth muscle.

Most of the sympathetic influence is vasoconstrictor and the neurotransmitter liberated from the postganglionic region of sympathetic nerves is noradrenaline. Sympathetic vasodilator fibers are present in the blood vessels of skeletal compartment and hence have role in increased blood flow through the muscles in the anticipatory response before the start of muscular exercise and also during muscular exercise.

Chemical factors (Table 8.1)

Other chemical substances, which can affect the peripheral resistance, are

Vasoconstrictor influence is by

- Noradrenaline
- Adrenaline when acts through α receptors

- 5 hydroxy tryptamine (5HT) or serotonin
- Vasopressin (ADH)
- Angiotensin II

Vasodilator influence is by

- Histamine
- Bradykinin
- Adrenaline when acts through β receptors

Table 8.1 Chemicals acting on vascular smooth muscle

Vasoconstrictors	Vasodilators
I. Noradrenaline	Bradykinin
II. Adrenaline	Histamine
III. 5. HT	Adrenaline
IV. Vasopressin	Adrenosine
V. Angiotensin II	Hypoxia ($\downarrow$pO$_2$)
	Hypercapnoea ($\uparrow$pCO$_2$)
	Lactic Acid
	Adenosine

Factors influencing peripheral resistance are many (Table 8.2). According to the following formula, resistance in general is affected by

$$R=\frac{8\,\eta\,l}{r^4}$$

8 = Integer of velocity of blood flow

η = *Viscosity of blood*

l = length of blood vessel

r = Radius of blood vessel (4th power of radius of blood vessel)

The length of blood vessel and viscosity of blood do not vary much easily in a normal person. Hence varying the radius of the blood vessel can bring about moment-to-moment alteration of peripheral resistance in the blood vessel. *The radius of blood vessel is under the constant influence of sympathetic nerves on the vascular smooth muscles of the arterioles.*

Table 8.2 Factors influencing peripheral resistance

I	Length of the blood vessel
II	Viscosity of the blood
III	Velocity of blood flow
IV	Radius of the blood vessel

VENOUS RETURN

Continuous return of blood to the atria/ventricles from respective circulations is called venous return. Generally venous return refers to returning of deoxygenated blood from peripheral parts of body to the right side of heart. The venous return is affected by many factors.

Factors affecting venous return (Table 8.3)

Table 8.3 Factors influencing venous return

I.	Pressure gradient
II.	Varieties of pumps
	• Skeletal muscle pump
	• Abdominal pump
	• Thoracic pump
III.	Vis-A-turgo
VI	Vis-A-fronte
IV.	Veno motor tone
V.	Extent to which the venous compartment is already filled
VI.	Drugs - Vene constrictor - noradrenaline
VII.	Presence of valves
VIII.	Gravity -

1. Pressure gradient

The pressure in the right atria (central venous pressure) into which the superior and inferior vena cavae open is around 0 mm Hg. In the peripheral veins the pressure is around 8 mm Hg and the pressure in the veins nearer to the heart goes on decreasing. In the right atrium the pressure (central venous pressure) is almost 0 mm Hg. So the gradient of pressure along the veins towards the right side of the heart is responsible for the flow of blood into right atrium. When central venous pressure becomes positive, the gradient is reduced and hence there will be decrease of venous return.

2. Vis a turgo

Is the force acting from behind. The contraction of the left ventricle creates a pressure that pushes blood from behind all along the vascular tree throughout the body. This pressure, which is getting created on left side of heart and which ultimately is responsible for pushing of blood from behind towards the right side of heart, is called Vis a turgo.

3. Vis a fronte

As stated earlier, the pressure in the right atrium is normally around 0 mm Hg. When the ventricles contract, the atrio ventricular ring is pulled down. As a result of this, the atria get expanded. This leads to creation of negative pressure in right atrium and the negative pressure is also created during sudden rush of blood from atria to ventricle. This is known as vis a fronte. This negative pressure exerts suction effect on the great veins and draws blood into the atrium.

4. Skeletal muscle pump

The veins are arranged in between the skeletal muscle fibres and are arranged parally. So when the muscle contracts the veins get squeezed. Due to the compressor effect of the muscle fibers on the vein, blood is made to flow through them. However blood is made to flow in the direction of the right side of heart due to the presence of valves in veins, which prevent back flow. If the skeletal muscles do not contract, there will be pooling of blood especially in the lower parts of body in the erect posture. This is because of two reasons namely

a. no activity of muscle pumps.

b. the gravitational force act as counter force for venous return and try to retain as much blood in the dependent parts of body.

5. Thoracic pump

During inspiration the intrapleural pressure becomes more negative. The contraction of diaphragm compresses the veins present in the abdominal region. A simultaneous increase of pressure in the abdomen and a more negative pressure in thorax, increase the pressure gradient for flow of blood towards the heart from the abdomen. Hence venous return is more during inspiration when compared to expiration phase during which the **intrapleural** pressure is less negative.

6. Abdominal pump

Normally veins present in the splanchnic region act as reservoir for blood. When the abdominal muscles contract, there will be increase of intraabdominal pressure and hence compression of veins occurs in the abdominal region. This increases venous return by increasing the gradient towards the thoracic cavity (heart).

7. Venomotor tone

The constant excitatory influence by sympathetic

nerves on the smooth muscle of veins is called venomotor tone. Because of this, the walls of the veins remain in a partially contracted state even under resting condition. When the venomotor tone is increased, the capacity of veins decreases. Hence they push more blood into the peripheral circulation from the reservoir compartment. This increases the venous return.

8. Gravity

As such the pressure in the veins is very less. When gravitational force acts on the lower parts of body especially in the erect posture, it will decrease the venous return from the lower limbs. If the person is in recumbent posture, gravitational force acts equally on all the parts of body, so there shall be better venous return.

CARDIAC MUSCLE

Heart is made up of cardiac muscle. It is striated muscle but involuntary in function. Unlike the skeletal muscle fibres, which are not branched, the cardiac muscle fibers are branched. There is presence of intercalated disc, which act as low resistant bridge. Through these discs the action potential can get passed on from one fiber to another. Hence cardiac muscle acts as a functional syncytium.

Properties of cardiac muscle are

- Excitability
- Autorhythmicity
- Conductivity
- Contractility
- Refractory period
- Distensibility

1. Excitability

Like the nerve or skeletal muscle, even cardiac muscle is in polarized state under resting conditions. The intracellular region is –90 mV when compared to extracellular part. When an appropriate strength of stimulus is applied there will be development of action potential. But unlike the action potential of nerve or skeletal muscle that is almost similar in configuration and ionic basis, the configuration and ionic basis of cardiac muscle action potential is entirely different.

2. Autorhythmicity

It is the ability of any tissue to generate its own impulse at regular intervals. The heart has this property. In a normal person the site of origin of impulse is generally the S-A node, which is also known as the pacemaker. In other words the rate at which the heart has to beat is predetermined by the frequency of impulse generated by this node.

When the *S-A node cannot act as a pace maker, some other parts like the A-V node or the ventricular musculature itself can act as pace maker. But the frequency of impulse generated by these regions will be less and the least being with ventricular muscle.* When the frequency of heart beating is as per the frequency of impulse generated by

- S-A node it is called as Sinus rhythm (60-90/min)
- A-V node it is called nodal rhythm (40-60/min)
- Ventricular muscle it is called idio ventricular rhythm (25-30/min).

The ability of the different parts of the heart to generate their own impulse and decremental frequency of impulse generation along the different tissues starting from the S A node can be demonstrated in an amphibian heart

by the application of Stannius ligatures I & II.

Special conducting system of human heart refers to (Fig. 8.2)

- S-A node
- A-V node
- Bundle of His
- Bundle branches
- Purkinje fibres.

S-A node is present in the right atrium near the opening of superior vena cava. This specialized region in the case of human beings act as pacemaker. The normal frequency of impulse generated by this region is about 60-90/minute (mean 75/min).

A-V node is present in the right atrium just by the side of interatrial septum in posterior aspect. The two different nodes (S-A and A-V nodes) are connected with each other through interatrial nodal fibres.

From bundle of His the bundle branches which take origin are present on either side of inter ventricular septum. Bundle of His takes origin from almost near the A-V ring and immediately branches to form right and left bundle branches. They form the connecting link between the A-V node and Purkinje fibres.

Purkinje fibres form the last part of the conducting system. They run deep in the ventricular muscle fibres.

The functions of the special conducting system are

a. Generation of action potential at regular intervals thereby acting as the pacemaker.

b. Conduction of action potential to different parts of the heart. The velocity of impulse

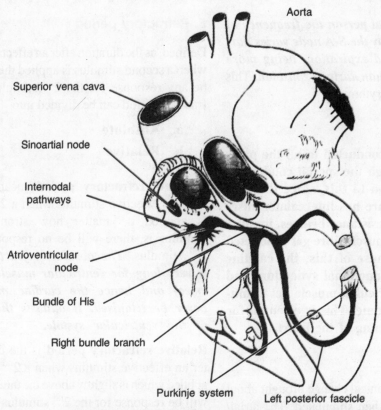

Aorta

Superior vena cava

Sinoartial node

Internodal
pathways

Atrioventricular
node

Bundle of His

Right bundle branch

Purkinje system

Left posterior fascicle

Fig. 8.2 Diagram showing special conducting system

conduction is fastest in Purkinje fibres (4-5 m/sec), moderate with Bundle of His and branches 1 m/sec) and least with nodes (0.05 m/sec)

c. Is responsible for the nodal delay at A-V node which ensures that the atria and ventricles will not contract simultaneously. This has to be taken care of, for ensuring the proper filling and pumping ability of the ventricle. The normal nodal delay is about 0.1 sec.

In the pacemaker region (SA node) the membrane potential is not fixed at any time. When membrane potential is around –60 mV, the efflux of potassium decreases, there will be slow influx of sodium and also of calcium due to the opening of T channels. Because of all these, the membrane potential gradually becomes less

negative and gives rise to the development of prepotential or pacemaker potential. When membrane potential reaches about –45mV, there will be opening of L channels through which there will be large influx of calcium ions, which leads to production of action potential in the S-A node. This action potential ultimately gets conducted to almost all parts of the cardiac muscle. Because of this S-A node acts as pacemaker in human heart.

The duration of the prepotential or generator potential to reach the firing level may be altered. When the parasympathetic nerve supplying the heart is stimulated the decrease in heart rate is because of the prolonged duration for the pacemaker potential to reach firing level and vice versa happens for an increase in heart rate when sympathetic nerve is stimulated.

Even in a normal person the frequency of impulse generated by the S-A node varies during inspiration and expiration, being more during inspiration than during expiration. This is known as sinus arrythmia.

3. Conductivity

The impulse gets conducted to all the parts of the heart through the special conducting system. In addition to this, since the ventricular muscle fibre has intercalated discs which act as low resistance bridges, impulse from one cardiac muscle fibre get conducted to the other. Because of this, the cardiac muscle acts as a functional syncytium and whole of the ventricular muscle get stimulated at the same time. This is essential for the proper functioning of the heart.

4. Contractility

It refers to the mechanical change brought about in cardiac muscle when stimulated. The atrial/ventricular contractile phase is known as systole and relaxation phase is known diastole. **The force of contraction can be altered by many factors like**

a. By altering the venous return, the initial length of the muscle fibre can be altered. As per Starling's law, which states that force of contraction is directly proportional to initial length of muscle fibres within physiological limit. *Varying the end diastolic volume can alter the initial length of ventricular muscle fibres. This effect is also known as preload effect.*

b. Sympathetic nerve stimulation or action of chemical substances (adrenaline), which imitate stimulation of sympathetic nerves will increase the force of contraction

c. Parasympathetic nerve stimulation decreases the force of contraction.

5. Refractory period

Defined, as the duration after an effective stimulus when a second stimulus is applied there shall not be any response for the 2nd stimulus. The refractory period can be divided into

a. **Absolute**

b. **Relative**

Absolute refractory period means duration after an effective stimulus when a 2nd stimulus is applied no matter how strong the 2nd stimulus is, there will be no response for the 2nd stimulus. *The absolute refractory period is very long for ventricular muscle (250-300 msec) and hence the cardiac muscle can never be tetanised. It outlasts the duration of the ventricular systole.*

Relative refractory period is the duration after an effective stimulus when a 2nd stimulus is applied which is slightly above the threshold; there will be response for the 2nd stimulus as well.

The whole of cardiac muscle obeys all or none law as the cardiac muscle act as functional syncytium. This facilitates generation of adequate force required for pumping of blood into the respective circulations. When ventricular muscle

Table 8.4. Properties of cardiac muscle in nut shell

i. Excitability	is effected by ionic concentration like K^+, Ca^{++}, Na^+
	Sympathetic and parasympathetic nerve stimulation and drugs
ii. Autorhythmicity	
iii. Conductivity	
iv. Contractility	
v. Absolute and relative refractory periods	
vi. Distensibility	

fibres get into fibrillation, there will be loss of the functional syncytium role of cardiac muscle and hence it leads to heart failure.

6. Distensibility

a. It refers to the extent to which heart can distend at the same venous pressure.

b. The chambers are covered by pericardium that limits the distensibility.

c. When fluid or blood gets accumulated in the pericardial cavity, the distensibility is restricted and hence force of contraction of the ventricle suffers.

CARDIAC CYCLE

Cardiac cycle refers to the sequential changes occurring during a heart beat. The heart normally beats at the rate of 75 times /min (mean value). So the duration of each heart beat is 0.8 sec, which is referred to as the duration of a cardiac cycle. Duration of the cardiac cycle can be calculated as follows

$$\text{Cardiac cycle duration} = \frac{\textbf{Time in seconds}}{\textbf{Heart beat/min}}$$

The cardiac cycle duration and heart beat frequency have an inverse relationship.

During a cardiac cycle the changes occurring in heart are

a. Electrical
b. Mechanical
c. Hemodynamic
d. Acoustic.

Electrical changes refer to the action potentials developing in different chambers like atria/ ventricles. The electrical changes are the prerequisites for any mechanical change in muscle.

Mechanical changes (Table 8.5) are nothing but the contraction and relaxation of the various chambers of heart. The atrial systole lasts for about 0.1 sec and diastole for 0.7 sec, whereas that of ventricular will be 0.3 sec and 0.5 sec respectively. However it should be noted that the atrial systole and ventricular systole shall never coincide normally, because of the nodal delay. Ventricular systole follows atrial systole and hence facilitates proper filling of ventricle. On the other hand, part of atrial and part of ventricular diastole can occur simultaneously.

Table 8.5 Events during cardiac cycle

Cardiac cycle (0.8 sec)	
a. Atrial cycle	
Systole 0.1 sec	
Diastole 0.7 sec.	
b. Ventricular cycle	
Systole 0.3 sec	
Diastole 0.5 sec.	
Mechanical Events	
a. Atrial -	
Systole	Volume change
	Pressure change
b. Ventricular	
Systole	Volume change
	Pressure change
Diastole	Volume change
	Pressure change

Unlike the atrial systole and diastole that do not have any sub phases, the ventricular events have sub phases.

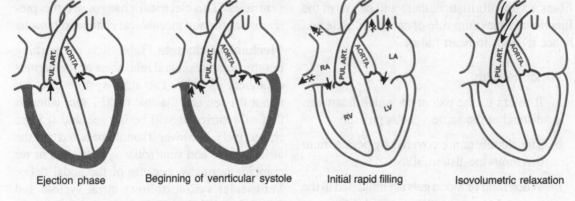

| Ejection phase | Beginning of venrticular systole | Initial rapid filling | Isovolumetric relaxation |

Fig 8.3 State of ventricles during different phases of cardiac cycle

Ventricular systole sub phases are

- Isovolumetric ventricular
  contraction (IVVC)   0.05 sec
- Maximum ejection phase   0.10 sec
- Reduced ejection phase.   0.15 sec

Ventricular diastole sub phases are

- Protodiastole   0.04 sec
- Isovolumetric ventricular
  relaxation (IVVR)   0.08 sec
- Initial rapid filling phase   0.10 sec
- Reduced filling
  phase/Diastasis   0.18 sec
- Final rapid filling phase/
  atrial systole.   0.10 sec

Due to the mechanical changes, the hemodynamic (pressure and volume changes in the chambers) and acoustic (heart sounds) changes also occur.

As the atrial contractions start, the pressure in the atria increase. So along the pressure gradient created by active contraction of the atrial muscle blood is pushed from atria into the ventricles. This usually lasts for about 0.1 sec. But hardly about 25% ventricular filling is because of active contraction of atrial musculature.

When the ventricular muscle fibres start contracting the pressure in ventricles will be more than the atria. *This may lead to regurgitation of blood from ventricles into atria, which is promptly prevented by closure of A-V valves. The closure of these valves is responsible for production of 1st heart sound.*

From the moment the A-V valves close, till the opening of semi lunar valves, the ventricle contracts as closed chamber. *So there will not be any change in the volume of blood present in the ventricle, but only the pressure increases.* Hence this phase is known as isovolumetric ventricular contraction (IVVC). It is important because during this phase a steep increase in pressure is builtup in ventricle within a short duration (Fig. 8.3).

When the ventricular pressure exceeds the diastolic pressure of aortic/pulmonary circulations, the semi lunar valves guarding the origin of aorta or pulmonary artery open. Now continued contraction of the ventricular muscle is responsible for pumping of blood into respective vessels. In the initial moments a lot of blood is pumped out and later on the volume ejected out is not much. The rise in pressure in the aorta/ pulmonary artery almost parallels the rise of pressure in the ventricle because these vessels act as damping vessels.

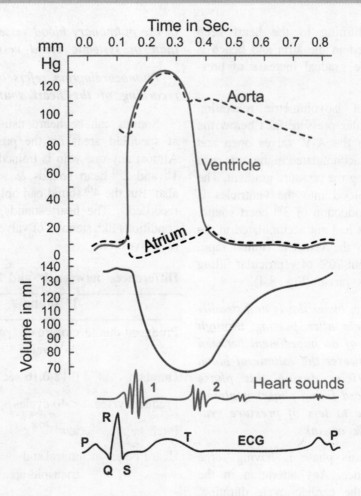

Fig. 8.4 Graph indicating the changes in heart during cardiac cycle

In the latter part of ventricular systole, pressure in ventricle start decreasing. At the beginning of the protodiastole, the ventricular pressure is less than the respective damping vessel pressure. *But still there is no regurgitation of blood into the ventricle inspite of semi lunar valves being kept open. This is because of momentum, the onward flowing blood continues to flow forward for sometime till the momemtum is broken (based on Newton's 1ˢᵗ law of motion).* By the end of protodiastole the momentum is lost and hence blood tries to flow back into the ventricle. This is prevented by closure of semi

lunar valves, which is responsible for the production of 2ⁿᵈ heart sound.

After the closure of semi lunar valves when the ventricles continue to relax as closed chambers because the A-V valves are yet to open. *So there will not be any alteration in the volume of blood in the ventricle but only a sharp fall in the pressure. Hence this phase is known as isovolumetric ventricular relaxation (IVVR).*

Throughout the ventricular systole and till the end of isovolumetric ventricular relaxation the A-V valves are in closed state. So the venous blood returning to the heart keep getting accumulated in the atria and hence is responsible for the gradual increase of pressure in atria.

At the end of isovolumetric relaxation phase, the ventricular pressure falls below the atrial pressure. So the A-V valves open and blood that had got accumulated in the atria rush into ventricles along the pressure gradient. The sudden rush of blood into the ventricles is responsible for production of 3rd heart sound. A lot of blood that had got accumulated in the atrium rushes into the ventricle (initial rapid filling phase). About 70% of ventricular filling occurs during this phase (Fig. 8.4).

After this phase, blood slowly and steadily enters the ventricle after passing through the atria because of no impediment between the chambers. However the volume of blood filling the ventricles during this phase (diastasis or reduced filling phase) is almost insignificant due to less of pressure gradients (hardly 3% or so).

But still diastasis phase is having some practical significance. Any alteration in the heart rate alters the cardiac cycle duration. This should not lead to undue over/under filling of the ventricle as the case may be. So by either prolonging or compromising the duration of diastasis, the ventricular filling is almost maintained for proper functioning of the heart.

Final rapid filling is nothing but further filling up of ventricles due to atrial contractions. This is the only part of ventricular filling that occurs due to the active contraction of the atrial muscle. *About 25% or so of the ventricular filling is due to this phase.*

Pressure changes in right and left side of the heart will not be the same during any cardiac cycle. In the right side of heart, the pressure is far less because the pressure

in the pulmonary blood vessels is much less than in systemic blood vessels.

Phonocardiogram refers to the graphical recording of the heart sounds.

Sounds can be heard using a stethoscope at specified areas on the precardial regions. Almost any one who is trained better can hear 1st and 2nd heart sounds & sometime the 3rd also. But the 4th sound can only be graphically recorded. The heart sounds get affected in conditions like stenosis of valves, incompetence of valves etc.

Differences between 1st and 2nd heart sound

	1st sound	2nd sound
Produced due to	closure of A-V valve	closure of S-L valve
Duration	0.12-0.16 sec	0.1-0.14 sec
Frequency/sec	< 40 cycles	> 40 cycles
Pitch	low	high
Heard better in	mitral and tricuspid areas	aortic and pulmonary areas
Indicates	beginning of ventricular systole	beginning of ventricular diastole

End diastolic volume (EDV) is the volume of blood in the ventricle at the end of diastole which is normally about 140 ml.

End systolic volume (ESV) *is volume of blood present in the ventricle at the end of systole and is about 70 ml.*

Stroke volume (SV) *is the volume of blood ejected out per ventricle per beat. Normal value is about 70 ml.*

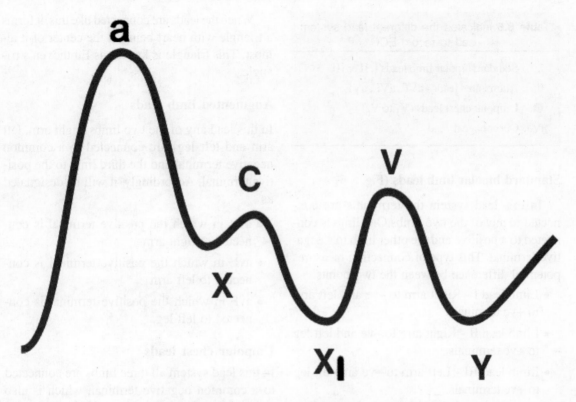

Fig. 8.5 Diagram showing jugular venous pulse

Pressure changes in atrium (jugular pressure change is almost similar) Fig. 8.5.

a is due to atrial systole.

a-**X** is due to relaxation of atrial muscle

c-indicates slight increase of pressure due to the bulging of valves into the atria at the onset of ventricular systole.

c-x_1 is because of the atrio ventricular ring being pulled down towards the apex of the heart during ventricular systole leading to drop of pressure in atria.

x_1-v gradual filling of atria throughout the ventricular systole and till the end of iso volumetric ventricular relaxation.

v-y is due to blood flowing from the atrium into the ventricle during initial rapid filling phase.

Electrocardiogram (ECG/EKG)

It is defined as the graphical recording of the summated electrical activity from the heart during a cardiac cycle.

Commonly used lead systems contain a pair of electrodes of which one is connected to a negative terminal and the other to the positive terminal.

• Standard bipolar limb leads (Table 8.6)

Unipolar leads are:

• Augmented limb leads

• Unipolar chest leads.

In any lead system there should be one electrode which is connected to positive and another to the negative terminal of a galvanometer.

Standard bipolar limb leads (Fig. 8.6)

In this lead system the terminals are connected to any of the two limbs. One limb is connected to a positive and the other limb to a negative terminal. This type of connection measures potential difference between the two points.

- Limb lead I - Right arm to –ve and left arm to +ve terminals.
- Limb lead II - Right arm to –ve and left leg to +ve terminals.
- Limb lead III - Left arm to –ve and left leg to +ve terminals.

When the leads are connected like this, it forms a triangle with heart being at the center of it almost. This triangle is known as Einthoven's triangle.

Augmented limb leads

In this lead any of the two limbs (right arm, left arm and left leg) are connected to a common negative terminal and the third limb to the positive terminal. Accordingly, it will be designated as

- avR in which the positive terminal is connected to right arm.
- avL in which the positive terminal is connected to left arm
- avF in which the positive terminal is connected to left leg.

Unipolar chest leads

In this lead system all three limbs are connected to a common negative terminal, which is also

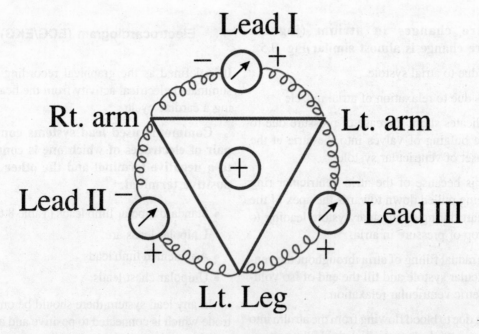

Fig 8.6 Diagram indicating the connections in standard bipolar limb leads

called as Wilson's central terminal. The positive terminal (exploring electrode) is placed on the chest at different places in the precardial regions. The designating of the lead in this system is based on the location of the positive terminal at different places.

- V_1- 4th intercostal place, on the right side just lateral to sternum.

- V_2- 4th intercostal place, on the left side just lateral to sternum.

- V_3- mid point between V_2 and V_4.

- V_4- 5th intercostal place on the left side ½" medial to mid clavicular line.

- V_5- 5th intercostal place on the left side in anterior axillary line.

- V_6- 5th intercostal place, on the left side in mid axillary line.

The configuration and amplitude of the waves recorded in the same individual differ with the lead system that has been considered for recording.

For all practical purposes of description the ECG recorded from the Standard bipolar limb lead II is taken into consideration.

Waves, intervals and segments and their characteristics (Fig. 8.7).

P wave

- Is due to the depolarization of the atria.
- Has amplitude of about 0.2 mV.
- Duration is about 0.08 sec.

Hypertrophy of atrial musculature results in increased amplitude of this wave.

QRS complex

Is due to depolarization of the ventricles. In this complex

- Q is due to depolarization of interventricular septum

- R is due to depolarisation ventricular musculature

- S is due to depolarization of base of heart and pulmonary conus.

- Has amplitude of 0.8-1.2 mV.

- Duration is about 0.08 sec.

Increase in the amplitude of this complex occurs in ventricular hypertrophy, which is seen in aortic/pulmonary stenosis.

Increase in the duration of the complex will be because of conduction blocks (bundle branch block).

T wave

- Is due to repolarisation of the ventricular musculature.
- Has an amplitude of 0.2-0.3 mV.
- Duration is about 0.3 sec.

P-Q/R interval

- **Time interval from the beginning of P wave to beginning of Q/R wave.**
- Normally the time interval is around 0.12 to 0.18 sec (mean 0.16 sec).
- It denotes the time required for the electrical impulse to reach ventricle from the SA node.
- When it exceeds 0.2 sec, it is concluded that there is conduction block.

Q-T interval

- Time interval from the beginning of Q wave to the end of T wave is called Q-T interval.
- Normal duration is about 0.35-0.43 sec.

P-R segment

- Is the isoelectric segment from the end of P wave to the beginning of QRS complex. During this segment whole of atria will be in the depolarized state and hence isoelectric.

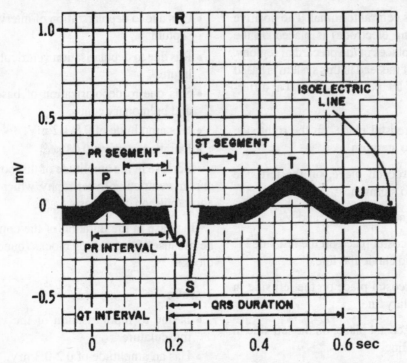

Fig 8.7 Diagram indicating the waves of ECG

S-T segment

- Is the part of ECG from the end of S wave to the beginning of T wave.
- During the segment the whole of the ventricles will be in depolarized state and hence isoelectric.
- Elevation or depression of this segment occurs in certain ionic imbalances in the body (e.g. hypo/hyper kalemia) or in myocardial infarction.

Significance of ECG (Table 8.7)

- **To ascertain any conduction blocks.** It can be complete or incomplete block. In complete heart block, the impulse from S-A node will not be able to get conducted. So the P wave will not be followed by QRS complex. After many P waves there may be one QRS complex. Now the QRS

complex appears because of idio ventricular rhythm. In incomplete heart block, the conduction time of the impulse from S-A node is delayed, which can be madeout in the prolonged P-R interval.

- **Any arrhythmias can be ascertained.**
- **Detection of myocardial infarction/ ischemia** with respect to the site, extent, duration and progress of infarction.
- **Relative size of different chambers** can be made out (atrial/ventricular hypertrophy is indicated with certain alteration in the amplitude of ECG).
- **Electrolyte imbalances** like hypo/hyper kalemia/calcemia result in certain changes in ECG.
- **Looking at the axis deviation** orientation of the heart can be made out.

Table 8.7 In nutshell uses of ECG

I.	To note the anatomical orientation of the heart a. Horizontal heart b. Vertical heart
II.	To find out the relative size of the cardiac chambers
III.	Abnormality in rhythm (arrhythmia and conduction (conduction block)
IV.	Detection of myocardial ischemia/infarction Location, extent, duration and progress
V.	ECF electrolyte lmbalance with respect to ECF - K^+ and Ca^{++}
VI.	Action of certain drugs - digitalis
VII.	To monitor moment to moment status of patient in post operative wards.

HEART RATE (HR)

The heart continues to beat all the time. The frequency of beats may vary. But under normal resting conditions it beats at 75/min (range 60-90/min).

When the heart rate is *above the normal range it is called tachycardia* which occurs in

Physiological conditions like

- Excitement
- Anger
- Muscular exercise
- Newborn infant.

Pathological conditions like

- Fever
- Thyrotoxicosis
- Hypovolemic shock.

When the heart rate is *below normal, it is known as bradycardia,* which occurs in

Physiological conditions like

- Sleep

Pathological conditions like

- Conduction blocks
- Hypothyroidism
- Complete heart blocks.

Nerve supply to heart (Fig. 8.8, 8.8(a)

Heart gets innervations from the autonomic nervous system.

Parasympathetic nerve supplying the heart is vagus. It takes origin from the dorsal motor nucleus of vagus present in the floor of the 4th ventricle in medulla oblongata. This nuclear region is also referred to as cardio inhibitory center (CIC). The preganglionic fibres synapse in ganglion present in the cardiac muscle. From these ganglia the postganglionic fibres take origin and supply the heart.

The right vagus supplies the S-A node, whereas the left vagus supplies the A-V node. Both at pre and postganglionic regions the neurotransmitter liberated by vagus is acetylcholine. At preganglionic region acetylcholine acts through nicotinic receptors and at postganglionic region it acts through the muscarinic receptors. *The muscarinic receptors activity can be blocked by atropine.*

Sympathetic fibres take origin from the lateral horn cells of T_1-T_5 segments of spinal cord. The preganglionic fibres synapse in the superior, middle and inferior cervical ganglia. The postganglionic fibres, which originate from these ganglia, reach the heart as superior and inferior cardiac nerves. The

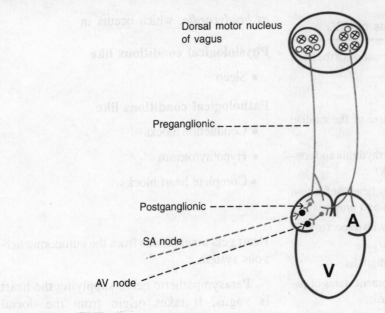

Fig 8.8 Parasympathetic nerve supply to heart

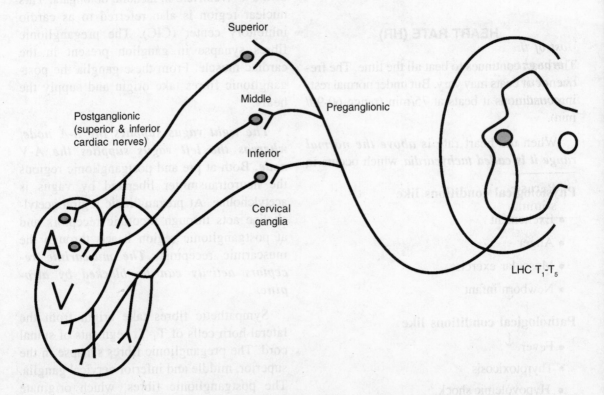

Fig 8.8(a) Sympathetic nerve supply to heart

neurotransmitter liberated at preganglionic region is acetylcholine that acts through the nicotinic receptors. *At the postganglionic region the neurotransmitter liberated is noradrenaline which acts through the beta adrenergic receptors.*

Heart rate is normally kept within the normal limits because of the balanced activity of the parasympathetic and sympathetic nerves action. *Even under normal resting conditions, there is some amount of constant inhibitory influence exerted by vagus. This is known as vagal tone. If bilateral vagotomy is done, the heart rate increases from 70 to 140 beats per minute even at rest.* Heart rate gets altered based on situations and activities in the body.

Regulation of heart rate

Most of the time the regulation of heart rate is brought about by the neural mechanism. The activity of the cardioinhibitory centre is constantly under the influence of the impulses coming from the following areas namely

- *Baroreceptors*
- *Chemoreceptors*
- *Joint receptors*

Regulation of heart rate by the baroreceptor mechanism (Fig. 8.9)

- Baroreceptors are present in the walls of carotid sinus and arch of aorta.

- Carotid sinus afferent nerve supply is by sinus nerve branch of IX cranial nerve and aortic arch is supplied by aortic nerve branch of X.

- Even under resting conditions there will be some amount of baroreceptor stimulation and hence impulses are being sent from these receptors to cardio inhibitory centre. These impulses exert an excitatory influence on the center.

Effect of stimulation of different nerves on cardiac functioning			
Parasympathetic stimulation	**Cardiac activity**	**Sympathetic stimulation**	**Tropic effect**
↓	Heart rate	↑	Chronotropic
↓	Force of contraction	↑	Inotropic
↓	Conduction velocity of impulse	↑	Dromotropic
↓	Excitability	↑	Bathmotropic

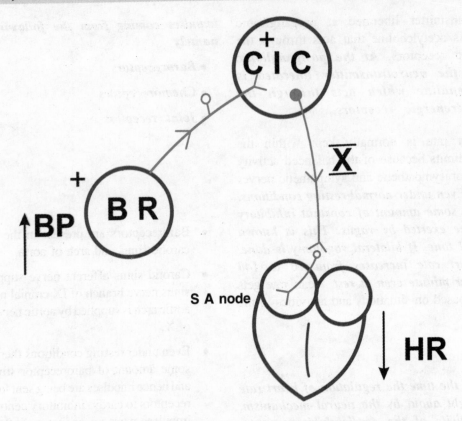

Fig 8.9 Diagram showing baroreceptor activity on regulation of heart rate

Increase of blood pressure	Increase in vagal tone
↓	↓
Increased stimulation of baroreceptors (receptor)	Decreased generation of impulse by pacemaker (effector organ)
↓	↓
More impulses along the sinoaortic nerves (afferent nerve)	Decrease of heart rate.
↓	
Increased stimulation of the cardioinhibitory center (center)	***Based on the above, Marey deduced a law, which states that heart rate is inversely pro-***
↓	

Table 8.8 Marey's law definition

Marey's Law states that the heart rate is inversely proportional to blood pressure i.e. increase of blood pressure decreases the heart rate

More inhibitory impulses along the vagus (efferent nerve)
↓

portional to blood pressure (Table 8.8). Exception for the law is in emotion conditions. An alteration in heart rate that is brought about due to stimulation of baroreceptors is known as Marey's reflex.

Bainbridge reflex

Distension of the great veins on the right atrium will bring about a reflex increase of heart rate. The receptors involved are the low pressure or volume receptors. The receptors are present in the wall of right side of the heart Both in the afferent and efferent pathway the nerve involved will be vagus and the center is cardio inhibitory center. *Hence this reflex will be an example for* the vagovagal reflex. The impulses from these receptors inhibit the activity of cardio inhibitory center to bring about an increase of the heart rate.

Chemoreceptor influence will be because of the receptors present in carotid and aortic bodies. When these receptors are stimulated, the afferent impulses go along the sino aortic nerves and exert inhibitory influence on cardio inhibitory center.

Cutaneous pain receptor stimulation increases heart rate and visceral pain receptor stimulation decreases the heart rate.

During muscular activity the movement of joints stimulate joint receptors and increase the heart rate. Impulses coming from the higher center will also contribute for the increase of heart rate in the anticipatory response.

Sinus arrhythmia is alteration in heart rate during inspiration and expiration. During inspiration increase in heart rate is due to Bain bridge reflex.

Apart from the neural mechanism, the other mechanism, which has influence on heart rate, will be hormonal mechanism. Hormones like thyroxin, adrenaline increase the heart rate. The direct effect of noradrenaline on heart is to increase the rate but since it also brings about an increase of blood pressure, there will be reflex bradycardia after few seconds due to increased stimulation of baroreceptors (Table 8.9).

Table 8.9 Factors regulating heart rate

1. Higher centre activity
2. Baroreceptors
3. Bainbridge reflex
4. Chemoreceptors
5. Joint receptors
6. Pain receptors
7. Circulating chemical substance like adrenaline

CARDIAC OUTPUT (CO)

Cardiac output is defined as the volume of blood pumped out per ventricle per minute. It is per ventricle because blood is pumped out from right ventricle to pulmonary circulation and from the left ventricle into the systemic circulation. From both the ventricles an identical volume is pumped out (Table. 8.10).

Normal cardiac output is about 5 l/ventricle/minute.

Body surface area and cardiac output have a direct relationship. Expression of car-

Table 8.10 Definition of cardiac output

Is the volume of blood pumped out per ventricle per mimute

Rt. vent. output = Lt. vent. output = 5 L. / min

Stroke volume is volume of blood pumped out per ventricle per beat

diac output in relation to body surface area is known as cardiac index.

Cardiac index = 3 l/sq m BSA/min.

Conditions in which cardiac output increased are (Table 8.11)

- Muscular exercise
- Excitement
- Fever
- Hyperthyroidism
- After meals
- Anemias.

Table 8.11 Factors increasing Cardiac output

- Muscular exercise (up to 700%)
- Anxiety and excitment (50-100%)
- High temperature
- Pregnancy
- Epinephrine

Conditions in which cardiac output decreases are

- Hemorrhagic shock
- Sleep
- Hypothyroidism

Methods for determination of cardiac output

- By Fick's principle
- Indicator method.
- Thermo dilution technique

Fick's principle

It states that the amount of a substance taken up or given out by an organ is equal to concentration difference of the substance in arterial and venous blood times blood flow through the organ per minute.

$$Q = (C_a - C_v) \times B \ F/min$$

Q = quantity of substance taken up or given out

C_a = is concentration of substance in arterial blood

C_v = is concentration of substance in venous blood

B_F = is blood flow through the organ.

While applying Fick's principle for determination of cardiac output it should be borne in mind that blood flow through the ventricular chamber in unit time is cardiac output. Normally the substance used is oxygen. While determining cardiac output by applying this principle, we will know

Q = volume of oxygen diffused into the body at lungs (250 ml/min)

C_a = arterial oxygen content (20 ml/100 ml of blood)

C_v = venous oxygen content (15 ml/100 ml of blood).

It should be noted that to determine the oxygen content in the venous blood the sample should be taken from the pulmonary artery, which is known as mixed venous sample. Venous blood sample from any peripheral vein cannot be taken because the venous blood oxygen content varies from place to place. A sample of mixed venous blood can be obtained by cardiac catherisation.

$$Q = (C_a - C_v) \times B_f \ (CO)$$

Rewriting the formula

$$B_f \ (CO) \times (C_a - C_v) = Q$$

So

$$CO = \frac{Q}{(C_a - C_v)} = \frac{250}{20-15} \times 100 = 5000 \ ml/min.$$

Dye technique

Most commonly used dye is T1824 or Evans blue because

- it gets mixed very easily
- it doesn't alter hemodynamics
- it is non-toxic.

Procedure

- Known amount of dye is injected through a peripheral vein.
- After every 3 seconds obtain a series of samples of blood from an artery to estimate the concentration of dye.
- After a gradual increase there will be a fall to startwith and a slight increase will be observed because of recirculation of the dye.
- Plot the concentration of dye against time axis on a semi log paper.
- Find out the mean concentration of dye.

Cardiac output can be calculated based on the formula

$$CO = \frac{\text{Amount of dye injected}}{\text{Mean concentration of dye}} \times \frac{60}{\text{time in seconds for one circulation}}$$

Table 8.12 List of methods to determine cardiac output
1. By using Fick's principle
2. Dye technique
Evans blue/T$_{1824}$
3. Thermodilution

Determinants of cardiac output are heart rate and stroke volume. Stroke volume is volume of blood pumped out per ventricle per beat.

So

$CO = HR \times SV = 72 \times 70 =$ approximately 5000 ml/min.

Regulation of cardiac output (Table 8.13)

Any factor, which affects the heart rate or stroke volume, certainly has a role in regulation of cardiac output.

Table 8.13 Factors regulating cardiac output
1. Venous return
2. Heart rate
3. Force of contraction
4. Peripheral resistance
5. Distensibility of the cardiac chambers

Heart rate

Any marginal variation in heart rate will not affect cardiac output. A gross variation of heart rate only alters cardiac output significantly. **But if the heart rate goes beyond 200 or so, there shall be severe decrease in ventricular filling time and cardiac output decreases.**

Heart rate can be affected by the stimulation of nerves. Parasympathetic nerve stimulation decreases the heart rate and hence cardiac output. Sympathetic nerves stimulation increases the heart rate and thereby increases the cardiac output.

Increase in heart rate and cardiac output can also be brought about by the action of hormones like

- **Thyroxine**
- **Catecholamines.**

Stroke volume

Stroke volume can be affected by

- Venous return — Preload effect
- Peripheral resistance — After load effect
- Myocardial contractility

Pre load is the load acting on the muscle even at rest and after load is the load acting on the muscle after the muscle starts contracting.

Venous return (Fig. 8.10 & Table 8.14) affects end diastolic volume and hence stroke volume. The mechanism involved will be

More venous return

↓

More ventricular filling and increase of end diastolic volume

↓

More stretching of ventricular muscle fiber

↓

Increase in force of contraction of ventricular muscle as per Starling's law

↓

Increased stroke volume and hence cardiac output.

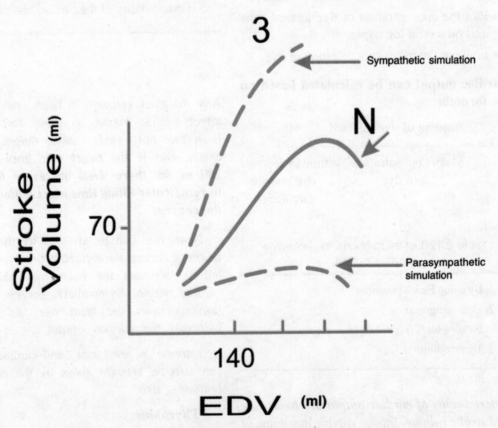

Fig. 8.10 Graph - venous return and SV with effect of nerve stimulation

Table 8.14 Mechanism of increased venous return increasing cardiac output
↑   Increased venous return
↑   End diastolic volume
↑   Initial length
↑   Force of contraction (As per Starling's law)
↑   Stroke volume - ↑C.O.

Myocardial contractility is influenced by (Table 8.15)

Stimulation of sympathetic and para sympathetic nerves. When the sympathetic nerve is stimulated there will be increase in stroke volume. The increase in stroke volume will be due to encroaching upon the end systolic volume.

Loss of myocardium (*myocardial infarction*) *decreases functional muscle mass.*

Circulating catecholamines *imitate the actions of sympathetic nerve stimulation.*

Hypoxia, hypercapnia and acidosis of myocardium *decreases contractility of the muscle.*

Pharmacological depressants (*verapamil*) *also decreases contractility of the muscle.*

Inotropic agents like digitalis increases contractility.

Intrinsic depression of heart also decreases stroke volume.

Peripheral resistance offered by the wall of blood vessels exert the after load effect. Increase of peripheral resistance leads to an increase in the diastolic blood pressure. Increase of diastolic blood pressure delays the opening of S-L valves during the systolic phase of ventricle. Due to this a lot of energy generated by the ventricles will be spent to overcome the peripheral resistance and to force open the S-L valves. Hence

Table 8.15 Factors influencing myocardial contractility

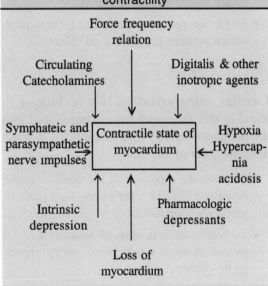

the residual energy of the ventricular muscle to pump out blood into respective circulation will be less. This decreases the stroke volume.

Muscular exercise and cardiac output

In severe muscular exercise cardiac output can be as much as 35 L/min. *The increase in cardiac output is because of so many factors like*

Heart rate increase will be due to

- Stimulation of sympathetic nerves
- Action of catecholamines
- Increased activity of joint receptors
- Increase of body temperature
- Bainbridge reflex.

Stroke volume increase will be due to

- Increase in venous return by increased activity of thoracic, abdominal and skeletal muscle pumps.
- Increase in venomotor tone.

- Action of sympathetic nerves and catecholamines on myocardial contractility
- Slight decrease of peripheral resistance, which reduces the after load effect.

Cardiac catheterization

Cardiac catheterization is a technique in which a thin tube (catheter) is introduced into the peripheral blood vessel and guided to reach different parts of the heart.

- To reach the right side of the heart it should be passed through a peripheral vein (anterograde catheterization)
- To reach the left side of heart it will be passed through a peripheral artery. (retrograde catheterization).

Advantages of cardiac catheterization will be to

- Measure pressure changes in different chambers of heart.
- Measure volume changes (ESV & EDV) in ventricular chambers.
- Obtain a sample of mixed venous blood.
- Study the septal defects.
- Introduce drugs directly into heart.
- Stimulate the pacemaker region.
- Record ECG directly from the heart.

BLOOD PRESSURE (BP)

Blood pressure is the lateral pressure exerted by blood on the walls of the blood vessels. *Blood pressure is measured by using the instrument* sphygmomanometer.

Systolic blood pressure is the maximum pressure recorded *in the arteries during ventricular systole. Normal range is 100 -140 mm Hg* & mean is 120 mm Hg in an adult.

Diastolic blood pressure is minimum pressure recorded *in the arteries during ventricular diastole. Range is 60-90 mm Hg and* mean is 80 mm Hg in an adult.

Pulse pressure *is difference between systolic and diastolic pressure. It is around 40 mm Hg.*

Mean arterial pressure is mean pressure exerted in the arterial compartment during a cardiac cycle.

It is diastolic pressure plus 1/3rd of pulse pressure (80 + 14= 94 mm Hg). – Table 8.16.

Mean arterial pressure is not an arithmetic mean of systolic and diastolic pressures because the duration of ventricular systole (0.3 sec) is less than that of diastole (0.5 sec). So there is inequality in the duration of maximum and minimum pressures and mean arterial pressure is always less than the arithmatic mean.

Mean arterial pressure is important as it determines the volume of blood flow through an organ or tissue.

Table 8.16 BP normal values

Pulse Pressure =
Systolic –Diastolic
120 – 80 = 40 mm of Hg
Mean Arterial BP =
Diastolic + $^1/_3$ rd of pulse pressure
= 80 + (13 or 14) = 94 mm of Hg

Measurement of blood pressure (Table 8.17) can be done by*Direct method in which a needle is inserted into an artery. This method is not practical in human beings, as the wall of the artery has to be pierced. This can be employed only when somebody is undergoing certain surgical procedures.*

Table 8.17 List of methods to determine BP

Measurement of BP

I. Direct - Inserting a needle into an artery

II. Indirect - sphygmomanometer

      < Palpatory method
         Auscultatory method

Table 8.18 Factors influencing BP

a. Age

b. Sex

c. Build

d. Posture

e. Emotions

f. Muscular Exercise

Indirect method is by using sphygmomano meter. *There are two different methods that can be employed using a sphygmomanometer. They are Palpatory method and Auscultatory method.*

In palpatory method an approximate systolic pressure is obtained whereas in auscultatory method an accurate systolic and diastolic pressure can be obtained.

While determination of blood pressure by auscultatory method the sounds heard using stethoscope are known as Korotkov's sound. They are produced due to the turbulence created by the flow of blood through the partially obstructed blood vessels. *In the normal course the blood flow through the blood vessels is laminar, the central most layer will be flowing at maximum velocity and the velocity of flow of the layers of blood that are more near to the wall of blood vessel get decreased gradually.*

Normally BP is expressed as $\dfrac{120}{80}$ mm Hg

Wherein the numerator indicates the systolic and denominator indicates diastolic pressures.

Factors influencing BP (Table 8.18)

Age

In newborn infants blood pressure is around 40 mm Hg. At about 12 years it is around 100 mm Hg and by about 20 years it is 120 mm Hg.

Sex

In females till menopause blood pressure is about 5 mm Hg less than the values in males. Beyond menopause it increases.

Build

In obese individuals it is more than normal.

Posture

In recumbent posture it is more than what it is in erect posture.

Muscular exercise

Generally there will be increase of systolic pressure and a slight fall of diastolic pressure.

Factors maintaining blood pressure (Table 8.19)

Table 8.19 Factors maintaining normal BP

1. Cardiac output
2. Peripheral resistance
3. Blood Volume
4. Viscosity of the blood
5. Elasticity of the blood vessels

Cardiac output and blood pressure have a direct relationship and cardiac output affects the systolic pressure.

Peripheral resistance and blood pressure also have direct relationship and peripheral resistance affects the mean arterial pressure.

Viscosity of blood and blood pressure also have direct relationship and this is going to affect the peripheral resistance and hence diastolic pressure.

Elasticity of blood vessels and blood pressure have an inverse relationship.

Blood volume when it is more, it can facilitate more venous return, which in turn increases cardiac output and hence increases systolic pressure.

Peripheral resistance is

$$R = \frac{8\eta, l}{r^4}$$

8 is the integer of velocity of flow

η is viscosity of blood

· l is length of blood vessel

r is radius of blood vessel

During moment-to-moment alterations of blood pressure among all the factors that are affecting the peripheral resistance, it is the radius of blood vessel, which can get altered easily and hence alters blood pressure.

The arterioles are the seat of maximum peripheral resistance as the smooth muscles are more in this region and they are under the influence of arteriolar tone exerted by sympathetic nerves.

Considering all the above factors, the final determinants of blood pressure are a) cardiac output and b) peripheral resistance.

Blood pressure = Cardiac output X Peripheral resistance

Regulation of blood pressure

It is very essential for a fine-tuning of normal blood pressure. During day-to-day life, there will be fluctuation in blood pressure for various reasons.

Altering the cardiac output or peripheral resistance or both, can bring about regulation of blood pressure. The various mechanisms operating in the body will bring about appropriate changes in any of these two determinants as the case may be, and bring about the regulation of blood pressure.

The centers that are involved in the regulation of blood pressure *are present in the reticular formation of brain stem. They are*

- **Vasomotor center (VMC)** that alters the smooth muscle activity of blood vessels by acting through the sympathetic nerves the details of which have already been explained along with peripheral resistance.

- **Cardio inhibitory center (CIC)** is also involved and it acts through the vagus nerve and more detailed explanation is found in nerve supply to heart and heart rate regulation.

- **Respiratory center (RC)** does contributes by bringing about a change in intrapleural pressure and hence affects venous return and cardiac output.

The various mechanisms involved in regulation of blood pressure can be grouped as

- Immediate mechanisms (Short term)
- Intermediate mechanisms.
- Long term mechanisms

Immediate mechanisms try to regulate the blood pressure within few seconds of alterations, whereas other mechanisms start acting only after few minutes to hours.

The various mechanisms involved in short term regulation of blood pressure are

- Baroreceptor
- Chemoreceptor
- CNS ischemic response.

Baroreceptor mechanism (Table 8.20)

- They start acting within few seconds.
- They are basically stretch receptors present in carotid sinus and arch of aorta.
- The afferent nerves that carry impulses from these receptor regions are sinus (branch of IX) and aortic (branch of X) nerves respectively.
- The operational range of these receptors is above 60 mm Hg mean arterial pressure.
- Even under normal resting conditions the mean arterial pressure is about 94 mm Hg. There will be some amount of stretching of the receptor areas and hence stimulation of the receptors.

Below 60 mm Hg pressure there will not be any stimulation of baroreceptors and above 180 mm Hg, the baroreceptors stimulation will not increase any more. Since the mean arterial pressure is 94 mm Hg in a normal person at rest, there will be impulse traffic along the sino aortic nerves. If there is sustained increase of blood pressure for prolonged duration, the baroreceptors get adapted to new pressure and hence fail to restore the blood pressure to the normal values.

The sino aortic nerve impulses will keep exerting some amount of influence on the following centers even under resting conditions:

- Inhibitory influence on vasomotor center
- Inhibitory influence on respiratory center
- Excitatory influence on cardio inhibitory center.

Table 8.20 List of the changes brought about during regulation of BP by baroreceptor mechanism

1. More number of inhibitory impulses to VMC.

• VMC is inhibited

↓ Vasoconstrictor impulses to arterioles ∴ Arteriolar dilation

↓ Peripheral resistance

↓ DBP

II. More number of excitatory impulses to CIC

*CIC is stimulated

Vagal tone increases

Heart rate gets decreased

Force of contraction decreases

Cardiac output is decreased.

Systolic blood pressure gets decreased.

III. More inhibitory impulses to respiratory center

*Inhibition of respiration leads to

↓ Venous return

↓ Stroke volume

↓ Cardiac output.

↓ Systolic blood pressure.

IV. Inhibition of VMC.

↓ Release of adrenaline and noradrenaline

↓ Cardiac output.

↓ Systolic blood pressure.

↓ Peripheral resistance.

↓ Diastolic blood pressure.

Baroreceptor mechanism of regulation of blood pressure is as per the Flowchart in the next page.

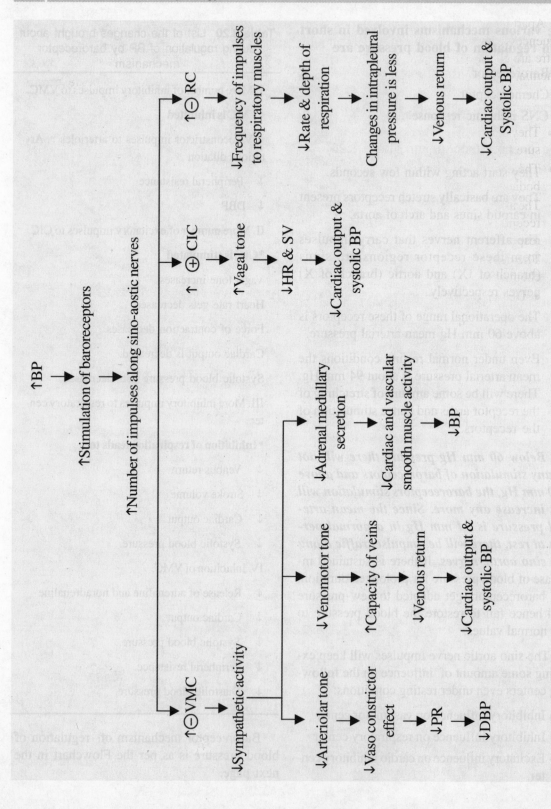

Apart from baroreceptors, some of the other influences which are acting on the vasomotor centre are chemoreceptors, hypothalamus, CNS ischemia, cutaneous pain etc. (Fig. 8.11).

Chemoreceptor mechanism

- They start acting only when the blood pressure falls below 60 mm Hg.
- The chemoreceptors are present in carotid bodies and aortic bodies.
- The afferent impulses are carried from these receptors by the sinus and aortic nerves respectively.
- The factors, which can stimulate the chemoreceptors, are
  - Decreased pO_2

- Increased H^+ concentration
- Increased pCO_2 in blood.

The afferent impulses from these receptor area reach brain stem and act on the centers. The influence of these impulses will be

- Stimulation of vasomotor center
- Stimulation of respiratory center
- Inhibition of cardio inhibitory center

PLEASE NOTE

The flowchart given for baroreceptor mechanism will be altered appropriately to increase blood pressure by chemoreceptor mechanism.

CNS ischemic response

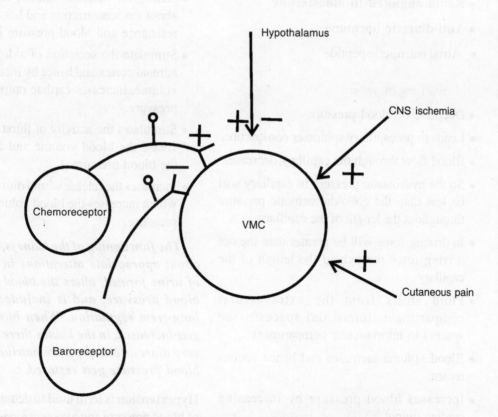

Fig. 8.11 Some of the factors influencing vasomotorcentre activity

When blood pressure falls below 40 mm Hg, there will be a severe decrease in blood flow (ischemia) to brain. This will increase the pCO$_2$ in the brain, which directly stimulates the vaso motor center. So the increased activity of the sympathetic nerves consequent to stimulation of vaso motor center will act on the vascular smooth muscles and cardiac muscle to restore both systolic and diastolic blood pressures.

This mechanism lasts for only few minutes. This mechanism is the last resort to restore blood pressure and blood flow to brain.

Intermediate mechanisms regulating blood pressure are

- **Fluid shift**
- **Renin angiotensin-aldosterone**
- **Anti-diuretic hormone**
- Atrial natriuretic peptide

Fluid shift mechanism

- Decrease of blood pressure
- Leads to precapillary sphincter constriction
- Blood flow through the capillary decreases
- So the hydrostatic pressure in capillary will be less than the colloidal osmotic pressure throughout the length of the capillary
- In driving force will be greater than the out driving force throughout the length of the capillary
- Fluid shifts from the extravascular compartment (interstitial spaces/tissue spaces) to intravascular compartment
- Blood volume increases and hence venous return.
- Increases blood pressure by increasing cardiac output.

Renin angiotensin mechanism

Renin secretion is from the juxta glomerular apparatus and the secretion is stimulated by

- Sympathetic stimulation
- Decreased blood flow through the kidneys
- Altered level of Na$^+$ in distal convoluted tubule.

Renin acts on angiotensinogen and converts it to angiotensin I.

This angiotensin I will be acted upon by converting enzyme and there will be formation of angiotensin II.

Angiotensin II helps in the restoration of blood pressure by

- Acting on vascular smooth muscle brings about vasoconstriction and hence peripheral resistance and blood pressure increase.
- Stimulate the secretion of aldosterone from adrenal cortex and hence by increasing blood volume, increases cardiac output and blood pressure.
- Stimulates the activity of thirst center to increase the blood volume and consequently the blood pressure.
- Increases the release of anti diuretic hormone which increases the blood volume and blood pressure.

The functioning of the kidneys, which bring about appropriate alterations in the volume of urine formed, alters the blood volume and blood pressure, and is included under the long-term regulation. When blood pressure gets increased, in the kidney there will be pressure diuresis and pressure natriuresis and the blood pressure gets restored.

Hypertension is term used to denote an increase of blood pressure and hypotension is for decrease of the same.

Hypertension occurs in conditions like

- Old age (known as essential hypertension)
- Hyperthyroidism
- Cushing's syndrome
- Conn's syndrome

Dangers of hypertension

- Ventricular hypertrophy
- Ischemic heart problem leading to myocardial infarction
- Congestive cardiac failure
- Cerebro vascular accidents
- Renal failure.

CARDIOVASCULAR SHOCK

The definition of shock will be a situation in which there will be generalised under perfusion of the tissues causing hypoxia. When there is imbalance between the circulating blood volume and capacity of blood vessels, it results in under perfusion of tissues.

Cardio vascular shock can be due to

- **Decrease in blood volume** (hypovolemic shock)

- *Depression of activity of either the vaso motor center or the lateral horn cells of spinal cord (as seen in stage of spinal shock after complete transection of spinal cord). In both the situations it leads to the development of* neurogenic shock.

- **Increase in capacity of blood vessels** (anaphylactic shock *is due to allergic reactions which bring about release of large quantity of histamine and* septic shock is due to toxins liberated by bacterial sepsis)

- **Left ventricular failure leads to** cardiogenic shock

What ever may be the reasons for shock, the decreased perfusion of tissues leads to development of shock.

Signs and symptoms of shock

- Decreased blood pressure
- Tachycardia
- Thready pulse
- Shallow respiration
- Cold clammy skin
- Cyanosis
- Sunken eyeballs
- Oliguria/anuria
- Loss of consciousness
- Thirst

In the initial stages of shock, the compensatory mechanisms try to restore the blood pressure and this is known as reversible stage.

During the reversible/compensatory stage the mechanisms, which try to restore blood pressure are

- Non-stimulation of baroreceptors and consequent alteration in activity of vasomotor, cardioinhibitory and respiratory centers.
- Chemoreceptors stimulation due to hypoxia and its activity on the afore mentioned centres
- Thirst reactions
- Anti-diuretic hormone secretion increases
- Renin angiotensin activity increase
- Fluid shift mechanism operates.

The above mechanisms try to increase the circulating blood volume and sympathetic activity (to increase the peripheral resistance) to restore the blood pressure.

When the compensatory mechanisms fail to restore the blood pressure, it progresses into the irreversible stage. The continued fall of blood pressure brings about further reduction of blood flow to the organs and the functioning of vital organs suffer. The situation may lead to death.

Special Senses

- Vision
- Chemical senses (Olfaction and gustation)
- Audition (Hearing)

Vision

Every individual has a pair of eyes. The perception of light through the eyes forms one of the important special sensations in human beings. Each eyeball has an optical system for image formation and also the neural mechanisms for converting these electromagnetic waves into the action potential so that information can be passed on to the central nervous system for perception.

The parts included in the optical system are (Fig. 9.1)

- **Iris**
- **Cornea**

- **Lens**
- **Aqueous humor**
- **Vitreous humor**

Neural component includes

- *Retina having the photoreceptors (cones and rods)*
- *Optic nerve and its pathway including cerebral cortex*

Differences between	Rods	Cones
Present	Not present in fovea centralis	At fovea centralis
Used for	Dim light vision	Bright light vision
Help for	Black and white vision	Colour vision
Visual acuity	Less	Maximum
Type of vision	Scotopic	Photopic

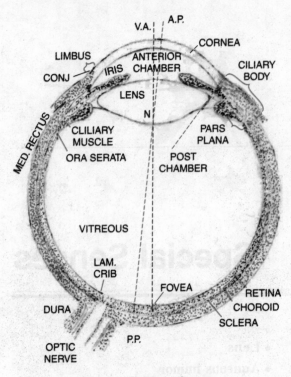

Fig 9.1 Section of eye

Aqueous humor

- Present in anterior and posterior chambers
- From the posterior chamber enters the anterior chamber through pupillary aperture
- Is secreted by ciliary processes
- Has Na^+, K^+, HCO_3^-, Vitamin C, Lactate, and Pyruvate.
- Drained into canal of Schlemn to enter scleral vein.

Functions

- Supplies oxygen and nutrition and removal of metabolic wastes and carbon dioxide from avascular structures like lens, cornea.
- It acts as a transparent media across which light rays can pass through to bring about image formation on retina.
- Helps to maintain intraocular pressure and hence the shape of eyeball.

Normal intraocular tension is about 15–20 mm Hg. When the pressure of the aqueous humor increases, it causes glaucoma.

Diopteric power of optic system

Total diopteric power is about 60D, of this the cornea contribution is $2/3^{rd}$ and $1/3^{rd}$ is by lens.

The corneal diopteric power is fixed, but the lens curvature can get altered depending on the situation, to either increase or decrease the diopteric power.

Field of vision

- It is the extent of the surrounding world that can be seen when the vision is fixed on a particular object.
- The different fields are
  a. Temporal
  b. Nasal
  c. Inferior
  d. Superior
- Of the four it is the temporal and nasal fields, which are referred to most often in visual field defects.
- Light rays from the nasal field falls on temporal ½ of retina and vice versa.
- In the visual field there is an island area of darkness, which is known as blind spot (optic disk). When the light rays fall on the optic disc that is devoid of photoreceptors the light rays can't be perceived. This is the blind spot.

Visual pathway (Fig. 9.2)

- Light rays get focused on retina and stimulate the photoreceptors.
- Impulses are carried by the optic nerve.
- At the optic chiasma the nasal ½ retina fibres of the both the sides cross over.

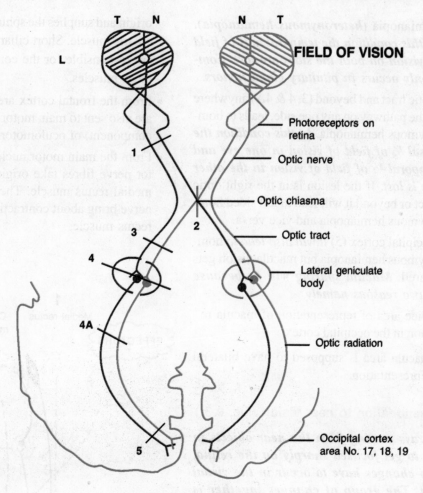

FIELD OF VISION

- Photoreceptors on retina
- Optic nerve
- Optic chiasma
- Optic tract
- Lateral geniculate body
- Optic radiation
- Occipital cortex area No. 17, 18, 19

Fig 9.2 Visual pathway

- Beyond the optic chaisma the pathway has, temporal ½ retina fibres from the same side eye and nasal ½ retina fibres from the opposite eye. This part of the pathway is known as optic tract.

- Optic tract fibres synapse in the lateral geniculate body of thalamus.

- From the lateral geniculate body the optic radiation or geniculocalcarine tract fibres take origin.

- They pass through the posterior limb of internal capsule.

- Synapse in occipital cortex area No. 17. This

is the primary visual area. Impulses are also relayed to area No.18 and 19. These areas are called visual association areas. They help in the analysis of color and other details of the image that is perceived.

Visual field defects (Fig. 9.2)

Field defects depend on the site of lesion in the optic pathway. If the lesion is at

- Optic nerve (1) *of any one side it leads to* complete blindness in the affected eye.

- Optic chiasma (2) *will lead to* bitemporal

hemianopia *(heteronymous hemianopia).* ***In this condition the temporal half of field of vision on both the sides are lost. Commonly occurs in pituitary gland tumors.***

- Optic tract and beyond (3, 4 & 4A) anywhere in the pathway on any one side, leads to homonymous hemianopia. ***In this condition the nasal ½ of field of vision in one eye and temporal ½ of field of vision in the other eye is lost.*** If the lesion is in the right optic tract or beyond it will lead to left sided homonymous hemianopia and vice versa.

- Occipital cortex (5) *it will also lead to* homonymous hemianopia but macula vision gets spared. ***Macula sparing will be because of two reasons namely***

   a.   wide area of representation of macula region in the occipital cortex

   b.   macula area is supposed to have bilateral representation.

Accommodation to near vision (Fig. 9.3)

Light rays coming from the near objects in order to get focused sharply on the retina, certain changes have to occur in the visual system. The group of changes together is known as accommodation to near vision.

When the photoreceptors are stimulated, impulses are sent to occipital cortex via the visual pathway as explained already.

- From the occipital cortex impulses are sent to frontal eye field area no. 8.

- This area plays an important role for accommodation.

- From this area impulses are sent to Edinger Westphal nucleus.

- From Edinger Westphal nucleus the oculomotor nerve fibres take origin and synapse in the ciliary ganglion.

- From ciliary ganglion short ciliary nerve takes

origin and supplies the sphincter pupillae and ciliaris muscle. Short ciliary nerve impulses are responsible for the contraction of these these muscles.

- From the frontal cortex area no. 8 impulses are also sent to main motor nucleus (somatic component) of oculomotor nerve.

- From the main motor nucleus the oculomotor nerve fibres take origin and supply the medial rectus muscle. The impulses in this nerve bring about contraction of the medial rectus muscle.

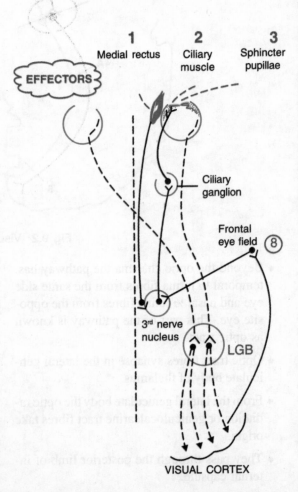

Fig 9.3 Pathway for accommodation

To summarise the changes and the purpose served by the changes are

1. Constriction of pupil

Constriction of pupil is brought about due to contraction of sphincter pupillae muscle.

a. Decreases the amount of light entering the eye.

b. Decreases chromatic and spherical aberrations.

c. Depth of focus increases.

2. Curvature of lens

Curvature of lens increase is brought about by the contraction of ciliaris muscle which leads to relaxation of suspensory ligaments.

⇑ **Diopteric power of lens (amplitude of accommodation)** *(Anterior curvature only shows further change in the curvature)*

3. Convergence of eyeballs

Convergence of eyeballs is due to contraction of medial rectus muscle.

Prevents diplopia or double vision by focussing the light rays on the corresponding points in two eyes.

Light reflex (Fig. 9.4)

It is the reflex constriction of the pupil that is brought about when a beam of light is thrown on the eye.

- Receptors are rods and cones.

- Afferent pathway is optic nerve, chiasma and optic tract.

- Centre is pretectal nucleus present in mid brain.

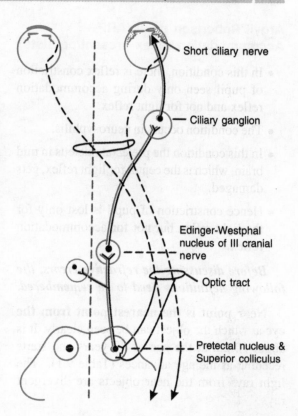

Fig 9.4 Pathway for light reflex

- Efferent pathway – Edinger Westphal nucleus, oculomotor nerve, ciliary ganglion and short ciliary nerve.

- Effector organ is sphincter pupillae muscle.

There are two types of light reflex namely

- **Direct** *in which light is thrown on to one eye and reflex constriction of pupil is looked for in the same eye.*

- **Indirect or consensual** *in which light is thrown on to one eye and constriction of pupil is observed for in the opposite eye. This is possible because the impulses from the pretectal nucleus of mid brain go to the Edinger Westphal nucleus of both the sides.*

Argyll Robertson pupil (ARP—Accommodation reflex present/persists)

- In this condition, there is reflex constriction of pupil seen only during accommodation reflex and not for light reflex.
- The condition occurs in neurosyphilis.
- In this condition the pretectal nucleus in mid brain, which is the center for light reflex, gets damaged.
- Hence constriction of pupil is lost only for the light reflex but not for accommodation reflex.

Before discussing the refractive errors, the following definitions need to be remembered.

Near point is the nearest point from the eye at which the object can be seen clearly. It is about 10 cm at the age of 20 years and starts receding as the age advances (Table 9.1). The light rays from the near objects are divergent rays.

Table 9.1 Near point and change in accommodating ability of lens with respect to age

Age (yrs)	Near point (cm)	Amplitude of accommodation
10	9	11-14
20	10	10
30	12.5	8
40	18	5-5
50	50	2
70	100	1

Far point is the farthest point from the eye at which the objects can be seen. It is at infinity. The light rays from the far objects are parallel rays. Parallel rays come from an object which is at a distance of 6 metres and beyond from the eyes.

Refractive errors of the eye are

Myopia (Fig. 9.5)

- It is also known as short sightedness.
- In this condition, the person can see near objects but not the far objects.
- The light rays from the far objects, which are parallel, get focussed in front of the retina.
- The condition is due to increase in the antero-posterior diameter of the eyeball.
- This can be corrected by biconcave lens that makes the parallel light rays to diverge before the rays strike the lens present in the eyeballs.

Hypermetropia (Fig. 9.6)

- It is also known as long sightedness.
- Person can see the distant object but not the near objects.
- It is due to decrease in the antero-posterior diameter of the eyeball. In this condition the reserve accommodative ability of the lens gets used up to see the far objects itself and hence not much of residual power of lens is left behind for accommodation to near vision. Due to constant strain on the muscle of the eyes, person suffers from headache.
- The light rays from the near objects, which are diverging, get focussed behind the retina.
- This can be corrected by biconvex lens, which makes the diverging rays coming from the nearby objects to get converged before they strike the lens present in the eyeballs.

Presbyopia

- It is due to decrease in the accommodative ability of lens as the age advances.
- Person's far vision will be normal but the near vision gets affected. The near point starts receding from the eye (Table 9.1).
- Because of the degenerative changes

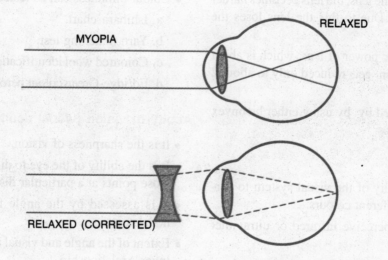

Fig 9.5 Diagram indicating refractive error in myopia with correction

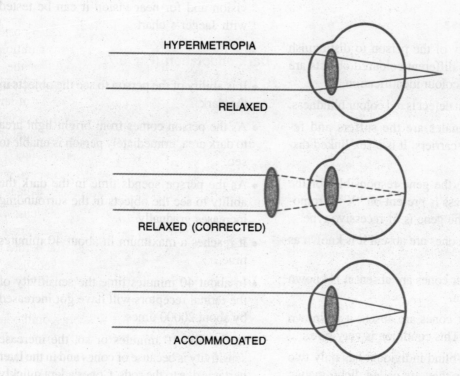

Fig 9.6 Diagram indicating refractive error in hypermetropia with correction

occusing in the lens, the lens becomes harder and thicker. Due to this the lens loses the elasticity.

- The diopteric power of lens, which is about 14 in children, gets reduced only to about 2 by old age.

- Can be treated by by using either biconvex or bifocal lens.

Colour vision .

- It is the ability of the visual system to perceive the different colours.

- Eyes can't perceive infrared or ultraviolet colours.

- Primary colours are blue, green and red.

- Cones are required for colour vision. There are three different types of cones for each of the primary colours.

Colour blindness

- Is the inability of the person to distinguish colours when different coloured objects are presented for colour identification.

- Most common defect is red colour blindness.

- More often males are the suffers and females are the carriers. It is a sex-linked disorder.

- It is because the gene responsible for the colour blindness is present on "X" chromosome. And the gene is of recessive type.

- If red colour cones are absent it is known as protonopia.

- If green colour cones are absent it is known as deutronopia.

- If blue colour cones are absent it is known as tritanopia. This condition is very rare.

- If any colour-blind individual has only two types of cones they are called dichromats.

- Monochromats have only one type of cones and are very rare.

- Colour blindness can be tested by
  a. Ishihara chart.
  b. Yarn matching test.
  c. Coloured wool identifications.
  d. Edridge-Green colour perception lantern.

Acuity of vision (visual acuity)

- It is the sharpness of vision.

- It is the ability of the eye to distinguish very close points at a particular distance.

- It is assessed by the angle formed at the nodal point.

- Extent of the angle and visual acuity have an inverse relationship.

- It is greatest at fovea centralis area, which has large concentration of cones.

- It can be tested using Snellen's chart for far vision and for near vision it can be tested with Jaeger's chart.

Dark adaptation (Fig. 9.7)

- It is ability of the person to see the objects in the dark.

- As the person comes from bright light area to dark area, immediately person is unable to see.

- As the person spends time in the dark the ability to see the objects in the surrounding increases gradually.

- It reaches a maximum in about 40 minutes time.

- In about 40 minutes time the sensitivity of the retinal receptors will have got increased by about 20000 times.

- In the first 10 minutes or so, the increase sensitivity is because of cones and in the later part it is due to the rods. Cones adapt quickly and for short time whereas the rods are slower to adapt but the action lasts long.

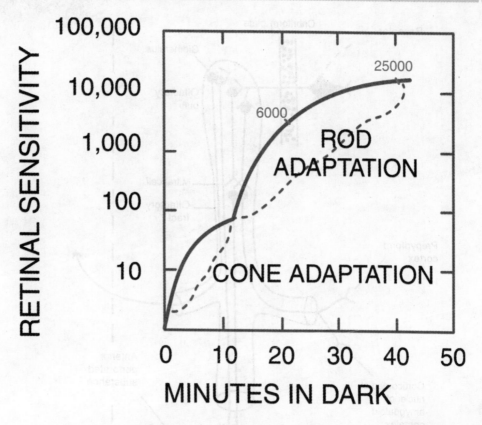

Fig 9.7 Dark adaptation curve

- It is due to the resynthesis of rhodopsin
- If a person is suffering from vitamin A deficiency, the person has difficulty to adapt at twilight. These persons are known to suffer from nyctalopia / night blindness.

CHEMICAL SENSES

- Smell (olfaction)
- Taste (gustation)

Sense of olfaction (smell)

- Is important for food seeking behavior.
- Has role in protecting the organism from the predators.
- Is important for sexual behavior in the animals.
- It is also associated with certain emotions and memories.

Depending on whether sense of olfaction is highly developed or not, the animal can be called as

- **Macrosmatic** which have very highly developed sense of olfaction e.g. dogs, ants.
- **Microsmatic** in whom the sense of olfaction is not developed much e.g. human beings.

Receptors for smell are present on olfactory epithelium in the roof of nose.

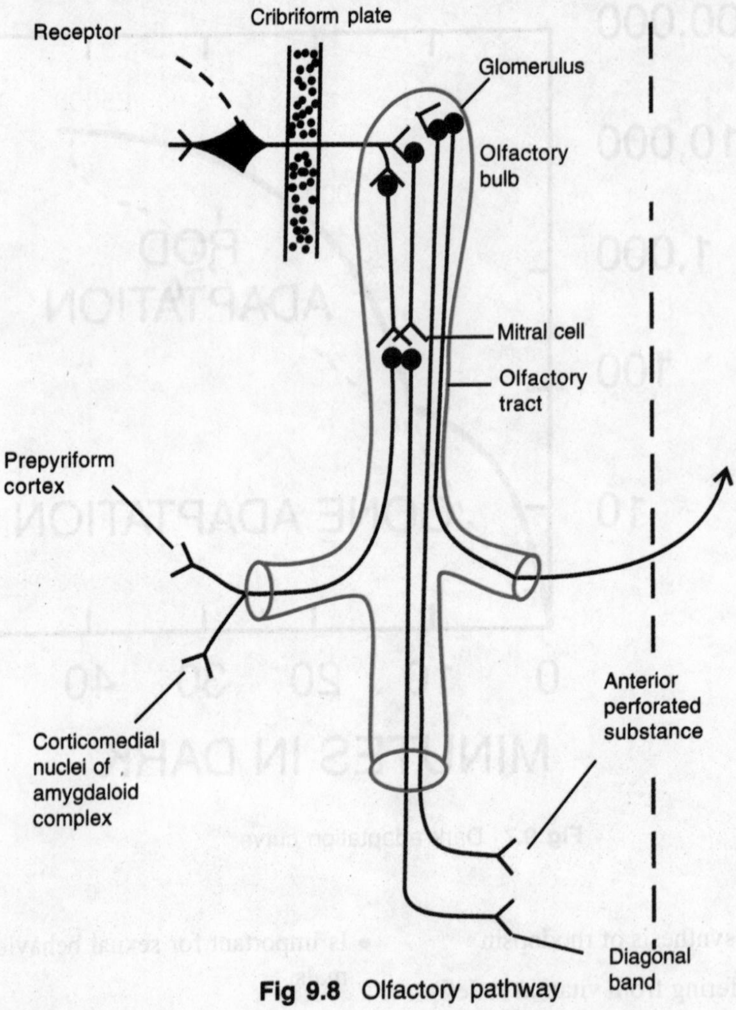

Fig 9.8 Olfactory pathway

Special features of olfactory pathway (Fig. 9.8)

- It is a short pathway.
- Thalamic radiation which is open to debate.
- There is no neocortical representation.
- **The receptors concerned with olfaction are the one which get adapted very fast.**

Anosmia means inability to perceive smell. Seen in common cold.

Parosmia means perverted sense of smell.

Hyposmia means decreased sense of smell.

SENSE OF TASTE (GUSTATION)

It is also a chemical sense.

Taste receptors are present in taste buds present in oral cavity (Fig. 9.9).

- *From the anterior 2/3rd of tongue the afferent nerve is chorda tympani branch of facial nerve.*
- *Posterior 1/3rd of tongue is glossopharyngeal nerve*
- *From the other parts of mouth it is vagus nerve.*

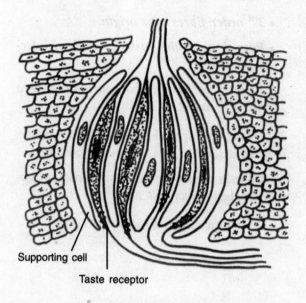

Supporting cell

Taste receptor

Fig 9.9 Diagram of taste bud

Primary taste sensations are four. They are

a. Sweet

b. Sour

c. Salt

d. Bitter.

● *Sweet is appreciated at the tip of the tongue, salts at sides in the anterior part, sour is also at sides in the posterior part and bitter is at the base of the tongue.*

The general sensations like touch etc. from the tongue is carried by trigeminal nerve (Fig. 9.10).

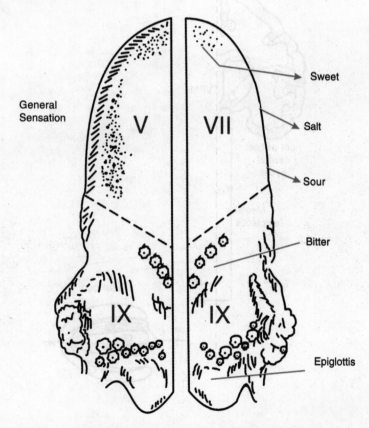

General Sensation

Sweet

Salt

Sour

Bitter

Epiglottis

Fig 9.10 Relative sensitivity of different parts of tongue for various taste sensations

Pathway for taste sensation (Fig. 9.11)

- *Stimulation of the taste receptors.*

- *Afferent impulses are carried by VII, IX and X cranial nerves.*

- *Relay in nucleus of tractus solitarius.*

- *2nd order fibres take origin.*

- *Cross the midline and ascend up as medial leminiscus. Now a days it is said the pathway is uncrossed and reach the ipsilateral cortex only.*

- *Fibres synapse in ventro postero medial nucleus of thalamus.*

- *3rd order fibres take origin.*

- *Pass through the posterior limb of internal capsule.*

- *Relay in the foot of post central gyrus area no. 3, 1 and 2.*

This is the only special sensation, which relates in general sensory area of cerebral cortex.

Ageusia means loss of taste sensation observed when person has fever.

Dysgeusia means difficulty to taste.

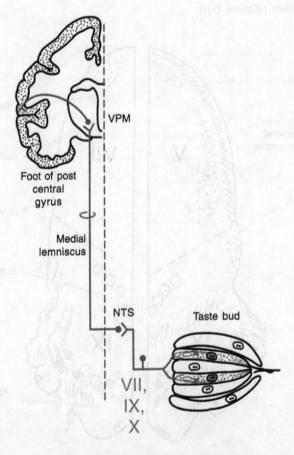

Fig 9.11 Diagram of pathway for taste

HEARING (AUDITION)

- Structure of ear
- Functions of middle ear
- Inner ear
- Auditory pathway
- Tests for hearing

The ear helps in the process of hearing. Ear is divisible into external, middle and internal ear.

- In the internal ear not only the structures concerned with hearing are present, vestibular apparatus, which is concerned with maintenance of posture and equilibrium is also present.

- The auditory receptors, which are present in the inner ear, convert the mechanical energy into electrical energy.

- The external and middle ear conduct the sound waves into the inner ear for stimulation of the receptors.

Physical characteristics of the sound

Frequency— determines the pitch of the sound (cycles/sec or Hz)

Intensity of the sound is determined by amplitude (dB). *This is nothing but the loudness of the sound. Sound intensities are expressed in terms of logarithm of the actual intensities.*

External ear

Pinna and auditory meatus are parts of this part. They help in receiving the sound waves and directing the waves towards the middle ear. The external ear helps to resonate the sound (resonance increases the sensitivity of hearing).

Middle ear (Fig. 9.12)

Contains 2 muscles namely
- **Tensor tympani**
- **Stapedius**

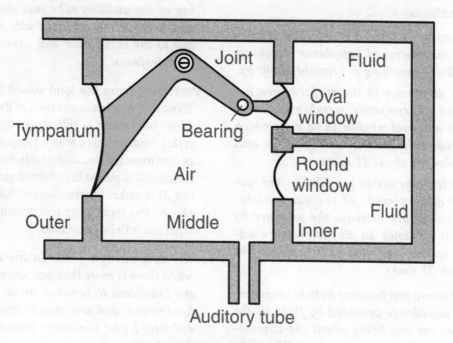

Fig 9.12 Diagram of middle ear

It also contains 3 ear ossicles namely

- **Malleus**
- **Incus**
- **Stapes**

In addition to the above, air is also present in the middle ear. The middle ear is separated from the external ear by tympanic membrane. It is connected to the pharynx through the auditory tube or Eustachian tube. The stapedius muscle attaches footplate of stapes to the oval window.

Functions of middle ear

Transmission of sound waves occurs from the external to internal ear through the ossicular system. *This is brought about by ear ossicles. Ossicular conduction has the ability to bring about* impedance matching. Impedance matching has to be brought about, as the sound waves from the air medium have to disturb the fluid medium in the inner ear for stimulation of auditory receptors. And fluid offers resistance for movement/disturbance.

The resistance offered by the fluid is overcome by the process of impedance matching.
1. *Impedance matching is brought about by*
   a. *The difference in the surface area between the tympanic membrane (66 sq mm) and oval window (3 sq mm) which increases the pressure acting on the oval window by about 17 times*
   b. *The leverage action provided by the special arrangement of the ear ossicles which further increase the pressure by about 1.3 times. In all the pressure acting on the oval window is increased by about 22 times.*

   The above mechanisms help to overcome the impedance provided by fluid in the inner ear and bring about the stimulation of auditory receptors in cochlea. The

fluid disturbance is essential to stimulate auditory receptors as they are mechanoreceptors.

2. Pressure equilibration on either side of tympanic membrane. *The pressure in the auditory meatus will act on the outer surface of tympanic membrane and is because of the air of the atmosphere. This pressure has to be matched by the air present in the middle ear for proper functioning of the tympanic membrane. The connection between the middle ear and the pharynx is through the auditory tube or Eustachian tube. Through this tube the air pressure in the middle ear can be altered either by facilitating the entry or exit of air into/out of the middle ear. Entry or exit of the air of the middle ear will help to match the pressure prevalent in the auditory meatus. Undue pushing or pulling of the tympanic membrane will cause pain and affects the hearing process as well. Act of swallowing can bring about opening of the auditory tube into the pharynx and help for movement of air. Any damage to the middle ear will cause conduction deafness.*

3. **Protection from the loud sound** is brought about by the reflex contraction of the muscles. When loud sound is anticipated there will be reflex contraction of tensor tympani and stapedius muscles. Because of this the tympanic membrane is pulled in and the stapes is pulled out. This makes the tympanic membrane taut. Due to this damage to the structures of the inner ear will be prevented.

4. Acts as a biologic filter. *In the ambience when there is more than one sound, it helps the individual to concentrate on the more loud sound and attention to that sound is enhanced and the other sounds are ignored.*

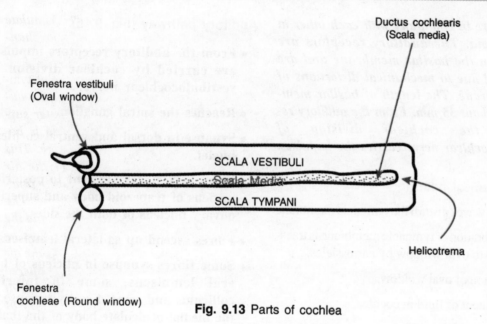

Fig. 9.13 Parts of cochlea

Labels: Fenestra vestibuli (Oval window) · Fenestra cochleae (Round window) · SCALA VESTIBULI · Scala Media · SCALA TYMPANI · Ductus cochlearis (Scala media) · Helicotrema

Inner ear (Fig. 9.13)

Structure concerned with hearing is cochlea. This contains the auditory receptors namely the organ of Corti. There are two different rows of hair cells in this part namely the outer and inner rows. *In the cochlea fluid is present. The cochlear region is divisible into 3 parts namely the*

- Scala vestibuli
- Scala media
- Scala tympani.

The scala vestibuli and media are separated by Reissner's membrane and scala media and scala tympani are separated by the basilar membrane. The organ of Corti is present on the basilar membrane in scala media (Fig. 9.14). The fluid present in scala vestibuli and tympani is called perilymph and in scala media it is endolymph.

Inner ear

As stated already the auditory receptors are

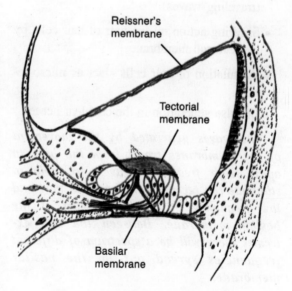

Fig 9.14 Structure of organ of Corti

Labels: Reissner's membrane · Tectorial membrane · Basilar membrane

present in cochlea. The various scalae have either the perilymph or endolymph. The composition of perilymph is similar to extracellular fluid and that of endolymph is identical to intracellular fluid. *Scala vestibuli and tympani are in continuity with each other at helicotrema. The auditory receptors are present on the basilar membrane and are stimulated due to mechanical distortions of the membrane. The length of basilar membrane is about 35 mm. From the auditory receptors the cochlear division of vestibulocochlear nerve carries the impulses.*

Mechanism of hearing

- Sound waves disturb the tympanic membrane
- The vibration of tympanic membrane is transmitted to oval window by ear ossicles.
- Vibration of oval window.
- Movement of fluid in cochlea.
- Membranes in cochlea move up and down (traveling waves).
- Shearing action on the hair of hair cells by the tectorial membrane.
- Stimulation of hair cells - act as micro levers.
- Impulse generation in the cochlear nerve.

The waves generated by the movement of the membranes travel from the base to apex. High frequency waves are able to stimulate the receptors in the basal part and low frequency in the apical part of the basilar membrane. Between the two extremes there will be a spectrum of different frequencies spread out on the basilar membrane.

Intensity discrimination of the sound is brought about by

- **Recruitment of receptors**
- **Based on Weber Fechner law**
  The details of the above are explained in chapter central nervous system (receptors)

Auditory pathway (Fig. 9.15)

- **From the auditory receptors impulses are carried by cochlear division of vestibulocochlear nerve.**
- **Reaches the spiral ganglion.**
- **Synapse in dorsal and ventral cochlear nuclei.**
- **From here fibres are sent to posterior nucleus of trapezoid body and superior olivary nucleus of both the sides.**
- **Fibres ascend up as lateral lemniscus.**
- **Some fibres synapse in nucleus of lateral lemniscus, some in inferior colliculus and some directly synapse in the medial geniculate body of the thalamus.**
- **Fibres from the nucleus of lateral lemniscus reach the inferior colliculus.**
- **From the inferior colliculus fibres reach the medial geniculate body.**
- **From the medial geniculate body the auditory radiation fibres take origin, pass through the posterior limb of internal capsule to reach cerebral cortex area no. 41 and 42 present in temporal cortex (primary auditory area). Auditory radiation fibres also send impulses to area no 21 and 22 in temporal cortex (auditory association area)**

Special features of auditory pathway

- **There can be as many as 6 order neurons in the pathway.**
- **Has bilateral representation.**
- **Crossing of fibres can occur at different levels (even at nucleus of lateral lemniscus and inferior colliculus).**
- **There are certain efferent inputs to the hair cells as well.**

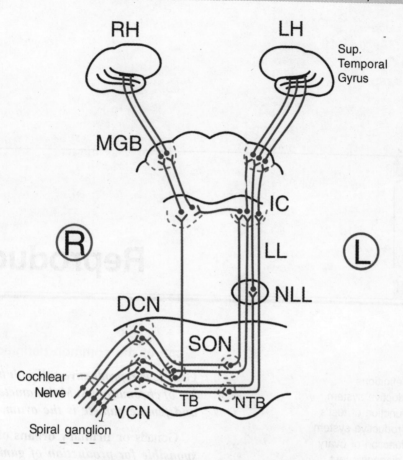

Fig 9.15 Details of the auditory pathway

Deafness

Deafness is the decreased ability or inability of the person to perceive sounds.

Types of deafness are

- Conduction deafness **occurs when there is damage to tympanic membrane, inflammation in the middle ear, accumulation of wax in auditory meatus. In such condition the bone conduction is better than air conduction.**

- Nerve deafness/sensory neural deafness/perception deafness **occurs when there is problem in the organ of Corti or any where along the auditory pathway. In this condition the air conduction will still be better than bone conduction.**

Tests for hearing

1. Tuning fork tests
   - Rinne's test
   - Weber's test
2. Audiometry.

10

CHAPTER

Reproduction

- Introduction
- Common definitions
- Male reproductive system
- Endocrine function of testis
- Female reproductive system
- Endocrine function of ovary
- Pregnancy diagnosis test.
- Placenta and functions
- Contraceptive methods

INTRODUCTION

Reproduction is the process of increasing the number of species or propagation of progeny. It is a process by which passage of genetic material occurs from one generation to the next, resulting in the formation of offspring having the characters of the species in general and certain characters of its own in particular. Chromosomes will be the carriers of the genetic materials.

Some of the common definitions

Gamete *is reproductive cell with haploid number of chromosomes. Male gamete is the sperm and female gamete is the ovum.*

Gonads **or primary organs of sex are responsible for production of gametes and act as endocrine organs as well. Gonad of male is testis and female is ovary.**

Fertilization *is fusion of male and female gametes.*

Implantation *is attachment of the fertilized ovum to the uterine wall.*

Accessory organs of sex *are necessary for reproduction but do not produce gametes. They help for the transport of the gametes. Accessory organs of sex in male are seminal vesicle, prostate gland, penis and in female they will be uterus, fallopian tube and vagina.*

Secondary sexual characteristics *are apparent features that differentiate the male and*

200

female. These characteristics develop at the time of puberty and continue in the rest of the period of life though late in life they undergo degenerative changes..

Puberty *is the stage or age of onset of the reproductive ability. In males it occurs around 10 to 13 years and in females it is between 8 and 13 years.*

Menarche *is the first menstrual bleeding in female at the onset of puberty.*

Menopause *is the last menstrual bleeding in the female, which occurs around 45 years. Beyond menopause the female loses the reproductive ability.*

MALE REPRODUCTIVE SYSTEM

The main parts included in the male reproductive system are as follows (Fig. 10.1) -

1. Pair of testis
2. Seminal vesicle
3. Prostate gland
4. Penis

Testis has both gametogenic and endocrine function *that is performed by different types of cells. Testis has three types of cells namely*

a. **germinal epithelium, which produces gametes (sperms)**

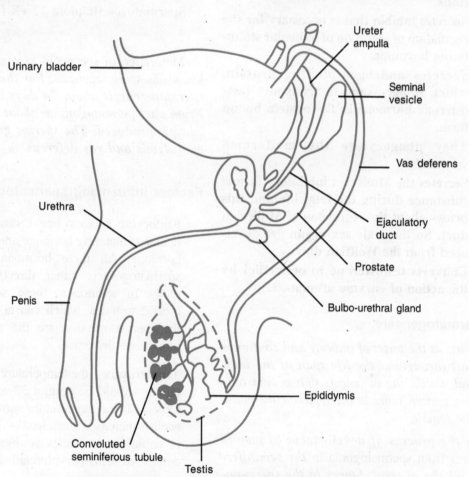

Fig 10.1 Parts of male reproductive system

b. Sertoli cells or supporting cell whose function is essential for proper gametogenesis.

c. Leydig cells have endocrine function (secretion of male sex hormone testosterone).

Functions of sertoli cells

- Nutritive function: the secretions of sertoli cells are rich in glycogen, which provides energy for the developing sperms.
- Contribute for the formation of blood testis barrier by the formation of tight junctions.
- Secretes inhibin that is necessary for the regulation of secretion of follicular stimulating hormone.
- Secretes androgen-binding protein, which is necessary to transport testosterone hormone in the protein bound form.
- They phagocytose the malformed sperms.
- Secretes the Mullerian inhibitory factor/substance during the fetal life and this brings about the regression of Mullerian duct. So the male sex organ get developed from the Wolffian duct.
- Converts testosterone to oestrediol by the action of enzyme aromatase.

Spermatogenesis

It starts at the onset of puberty and continues almost throughout the life span of the individual, unlike the oogenesis that occurs only during certain years in the reproductive phase of the female.

It is the process of development of mature sperms from spermatogonia *in the seminiferous tubules of testis. Stages in the spermatogenesis are*

Spermatogonia (diploid 22 pairs + X,Y)

↓ Mitosis

Primary spermatocyte (diploid 22 pairs + X,Y)

↓ Meiotic division

Secondary spermatocyte (haploid 22 +X / 22 + Y)

↓ Meiotic division

Spermatid (haploid 22 +X / 22 + Y)

↓

Spermatozoa (haploid 22 +X / 22 + Y)

Maturation of spermatid to spermatozoa is known as spermiogenesis. *For the process of spermatogenesis about 74 days is required. From one spermatogonium about 512 sperms can get produced. The sperms get stored in epidydymis and vas deferens.*

Factors influencing spermatogenesis

- **Endocrine factors** like testosterone, follicular stimulating hormone and leutinizing hormone. All these hormone affect the spermatogenesis either directly or indirectly. In addition to these, some of the other hormones, which can also influence the spermatogenesis are the growth hormone and thyroxine.

- **Temperature**—the temperature in the scrotal sac should be around 32 to 35 degree Celsius. If the temperature surrounding the testis is increased it can lead to degeneration of seminiferous tubules as observed in undescended testis (Cryptorchidism).

- **Nutritional factors** like certain vitamins.

- **Inhibiting factors** like
  - radiation
  - alcohol
  - nicotine
  - infections (mumps)

  which can lead to sterility.

Cryptorchidism

In this condition the testis remains in the abdomen. *In the intrauterine life testis develop in abdomen and around 7th month of intrauterine life they descend into scrotal sacs. If they continue to remain in the abdomen the temperature which is more in abdomen region brings about the degeneration of seminiferous tubules. So the sperm production gets affected.* The person becomes sterile. *Endocrine function of the Leydig cells continues and hence testosterone level remains normal.*

Endocrine function of testis

The sex hormone of male is testosterone and is secreted by testis.

Actions

During fetal life

- **Responsible for the descent of testis into the scrotal sac.**
- **Development of male external and internal genitalia.**
- **Development of male brain (hypothalamus) which is concerned with secretion of follicular stimulating hormone and leutinizing hormone. In males the secretion of the above two hormones will not have any cyclical change in 28 days, unlike what is observed in females.**

Table 10.1 Body changes at puberty in boys
1. External genitalia
2. Internal genitalia
3. Voice
4. Mental
5. Body conformation
6. Skin
7. Hair growth

Table 10.2 List of actions of testosterone
• Gametogenesis (Spermatogenesis)
• Development of male secondary sexual charecteristics and maintenance of some of them
• Maintenance of size of prostate and seminal vesicle.
• On anterior pituitary to regulate secretion of gonadotropic hormones
• Anabolic and growth promoting effects
• Actions during foetal stage of development

At the onset of puberty (Table 10.1.& 10.2)

- **Initiates spermatogenesis.**
- **Responsible for growth of accessory organs of sex.**
- **Brings about the development of secondary sexual characteristics like** (Table 10.1)

  a. *Growth of beard and mustache*

  b. *Development of hair in pubic and axillary regions*

  c. *Aggressive nature of male*

  d. *Broad shoulder and narrow hip*

  e. *Voice becoming more deep*

  f. *Receding of frontal hair line*

  g. *Increase of muscle mass*

  h. *Development of libido.*

- **Increases the protein anabolism and hence more muscle development and chondrogenesis and collagen synthesis.**
- **Promotes early fusion of epiphyseal plates which now a days they say is because of estrogen.**
- **Increases production of erythrocytes.**
- **Exerts negative feedback control over the anterior pituitary gland on the se-** cretion of gonadotropic hormones (Fig. 10.2).

During rest of life

- **Maintenance of spermatogenesis.**
- **Maintenance of accessory organs of sex.**
- **Maintenance of negative feed back over the anterior pituitary gland over follicular stimulating and leutinising hormone secretions.**

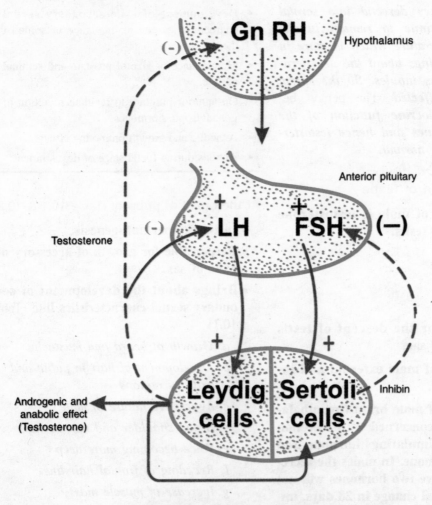

Fig 10.2 Regulation of secretion of hormones

Semen (Table 10.3)

- **Quantity is about 2 to 5 ml/ejaculation.**
- **% Contribution is —**
  - **a. 10% spermatozoa**
  - **b. 60% is secretions of seminal vesicle**
  - **c. 30% is prostatic secretion.**
- **pH 7.4**

Normal sperm count is about 40–100 million/ml. Sperm count is less when the frequency of ejaculation is more. If the count is less than 50% of normal the person becomes infertile and below 20%, fertility gets affected severely.

Table 10.3 Details of composition of semen and sperms	
Quantity*	2 -- 5 ml/ejaculate
pH	7.4
about <10%	Spermatozoa
about 30%	Prostatic Secretion
about 60%	Seminal vesicle secretion
Spermatozoa	
<10% of semen	
40-100 million/ml	
Survival period in the female genital tract is 24-72 hours	
Do not survive in acid medium	
* Variable - ↓ with repeated ejaculation	

Oligospermia is the decreased sperm count and azoospermia is absence of sperms.

Sperms survive in the female genital tract for about 48–72 hours. Acidic medium is hostile for survival. In the laboratory conditions at 4 degree Celsius they survive for about few weeks, whereas at minus 70 degree Celsius they can survive for years.

Composition of secretion of

a. Seminal vesicle is

- Fructose
- Ascorbic acid
- Prostaglandins
- Fibrinogen
- Flavin compounds.

b. Prostate gland is

- Citric acid
- Fibrinolysin
- Calcium
- Spermine.

Vasectomy

- *It is cutting and ligating of vas deferens of either side.*
- *It is the permanent method of family planning (contraception) in male. After vasectomy, ejaculation of semen still occurs as 90% of semen is due to secretions from seminal vesicle and prostate gland. So the volume of semen does not get affected much but sperms will be absent in semen. The person becomes sterile (Table 10.4).*
- After vasectomy the person has to be careful for the next two months or so, as the sperms that have got stored already in the ampulla of vas can still get ejaculated along with semen and lead to conception.

Orchidectomy *means removal of testis or castration. Effects of orchidectomy before and after puberty are*

Before puberty

- No testosterone secretion and hence no growth of accessory organs of sex and development of secondary sexual characteristics.

- No onset of puberty
- Overall growth of body decreases
- Voice remains high pitched
- Body configuration almost like female
- Absence of libido and the person becomes impotent.

After puberty (Table 10.4)

- No spermatogenesis
- Skeletal growth that had occured earlier will remain the same.
- Person becomes sterile
- Accessory organs of sex remain normal, but the glands like seminal vesicle and prostate undergo atrophy.

- Libido may be normal.

Tests for male infertility

Semen analysis for

- **Volume**
- **pH**
- **Sperm count**
- **Morphology of sperms**
- **Motility.**
- **Testicular biopsy.**
- **Hormonal assay—Follicular stimulating hormone, leutinizing hormone and testosterone levels in circulation are estimated.**

Table 10.4 Differences in the features between bilateral vasectomy, cryptorchidism and castration after puberty in a male

Features	Vasectomy	Cryptorchidism	Castration
1. Ejaculation of semen	N	N	↓↓↓
2. Semen volume	N	N	↓↓↓
3. Semen composition. (sperms)	←	Sperms absent	→
4. Fertility	←	Infertile	→
5. Testosterone production	N	N	Nil
6. Accessory glands	N	N	Regress
7. Secondary sexual characters	N	N	N
8. Libido	N	N	N/↓

FEMALE REPRODUCTIVE SYSTEM

The important parts in the female reproductive system are (Fig. 10.3)

1. Pair of ovaries
2. Fallopian tubes
3. Uterus
4. Vagina

The primary organ of sex in female is ovary, which has got both the gametogenic and endocrine function. The sex hormones of female are estrogen and progesterone. *The hormones are secreted in a cyclical fashion throughout the reproductive phase in females. During each cycle there will be growth and maturation of an ovum from any one of the ovaries. In case there is no fertilization the onset of next men-*

strual cycle prepares the female reproductive system to undergo the cyclical changes again.

Menstrual cycle

The cyclical changes will be taking place in the

    a. Ovary

    b. Uterus

    c. Cervix

    d. Vagina

- **In 28 days normally.**
- **And the duration of the cycle is not fixed.**
- **Duration can be as little as 20 days and as many as 45 days.**

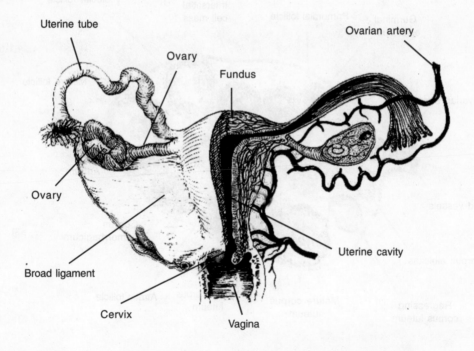

Figure 10.3 Parts of female reproductive system

Counting of the days in a cycle begins on the day the menstruation starts.

- **The menstrual discharge contains blood, damaged endometrial cells, damaged endometrial glands and endothelial cells of damaged blood vessels.**

During any menstrual cycle the changes will be taking place simultaneously in the

a. Ovary termed as ovarian cycle

b. Uterus termed as uterine or endome trial cycle

c. Vagina termed as vaginal cycle.

Oogenesis is the growth and maturation of an ovum. *It occurs in any one of the ovaries during any menstrual cycle. The number of oogonia is fixed at birth.*

Stages in oogenesis

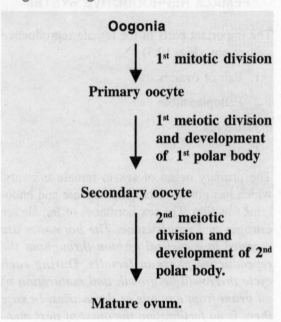

Oogonia

↓ 1st mitotic division

Primary oocyte

↓ 1st meiotic division and development of 1st polar body

Secondary oocyte

↓ 2nd meiotic division and development of 2nd polar body.

Mature ovum.

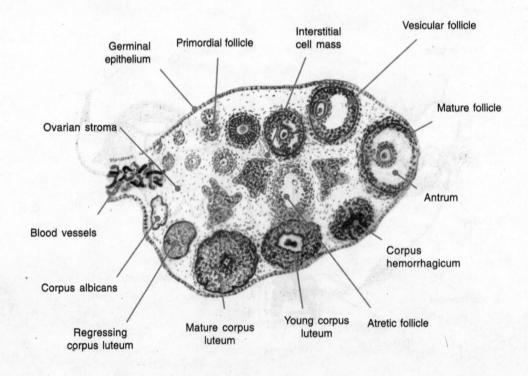

Figure 10.3(a) Changes in ovary during a menstrual cycle

Ovarian cycle Fig. 10.3(a)

Formation of primordial follicles begins around the 8th week of intrauterine life.

About 1 million follicles are present at birth.

Due to atresia, by the time of onset of puberty there will be only about 300000 follicles of which only around 400 get matured into ova.

The different stages of ovarian cycle are

- **Follicular phase**
- **Luteal phase**

Follicular phase

- Under the influence of the hormone FSH secreted from the anterior pituitary gland about 5 to 6 follicles start developing.
- Of which only one of follicles grows further and matures. This follicle is known as dominant follicle.
- The remaining follicles start regressing. They are termed as the atretic follicles.
- One of the follicles, which is maturing, develops a cavity and the cavity is known as antrum.
- As the follicle is maturing the size of the cavity increases and the fluid start accumulating in the cavity.
- All these changes are brought about due to the action of follicular stimulating hormone of anterior pituitary gland and the estrogen secreted by the theca interna cells of the maturing follicle.
- Around the 14th day in a 28 day menstrual cycle, ovum is liberated from the mature follicle. This process is known as ovulation. The fimbriated ends of the fallopian tubes pick up the released ovum from the abdominal cavity.

- The hormone, which is responsible for the ovulation, is leutinizing hormone surge, which is brought about by the positive feedback regulation exerted by estrogen.

Luteal phase

- The cavity of the follicle, which has released the ovum, gets filled with blood.
- This is known as corpus hemorragicum.
- Around the 16th day the blood spots are replaced by lipid rich luteal cells and hence it is known as corpus luteum.
- The corpus luteum starts secreting estrogen and progesterone till around 24th day.
- In case there is no fertilization the corpus luteum starts regressing (leuteolysis) and around the 28th day there will be formation of corpus albicans.

Uterine cycle–Phases are (Fig. 10.4)

- **Menstrual**
- **Proliferative**
- **Secretory**

Menstrual phase

Menstrual bleeding lasts for about 3 to 5 days. The counting of the day of the cycle start from the day the bleeding starts.

Proliferative phase

Is from the day 5 to day 14. The duration of this phase is not fixed. It can get shortened or prolonged depending on the number of days the particular menstrual cycle lasts. This phase corresponds to the follicular phase of ovarian cycle.

Changes brought about in the uterus/ endometrium are

- **Thickness of the endometrium, which**

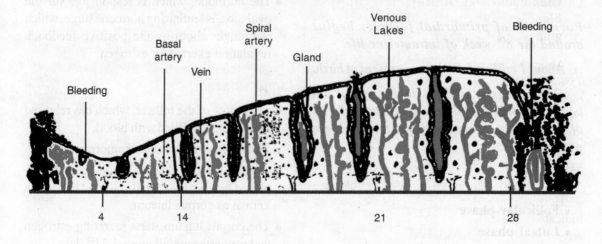

Figure 10.4 Changes in uterus during a menstrual cycle

was less than 2 mm at the cessation of bleeding, increases to about 4 to 5 mm. This is due to multiplication of the cells by mitotic cell division.

- Uterine glands and ducts grow but donot start secreting.

- Spiral arteries also start developing.

For all the above changes to be brought about in the endometrium, the hormone responsible is estrogen which is secreted by the theca interna cells of the maturing follicle.

Secretory phase

This phase lasts for about 14 days. The duration of this phase is very much fixed irrespective of the duration of the menstrual cycle. *This phase corresponds to the luteal phase of the ovarian cycle.*

Changes occurring during this phase are

- Endometrium gets thickened further and blood supply increases.

- Ducts of the uterine glands become more coiled.

- Spiral arteries also become more tortuous.

- Uterine glands start secreting. These secretions are rich in glycogen which is necessary to supply nutrition.

- Veins develop and venous lakes appear.

- Endometrium becomes edematous.

All these changes are due to the influence of the hormones estrogen and progesterone that are secreted by the corpus luteum. *In case there is no fertilization of the ovum, the degeneration of the corpus luteum leads to loss of the hormonal support to the endometrium. This results in*

- Spasm of the spiral arteries for few hours and the endothelial lining of the arteries above the spasm get damaged due to ischemia.

- Shrinking of the endometrium and necrosis of the endometrium above the level of spasm.

After few hours when the spasm is released, since the endothelial lining and endometrial region have got damaged, blood gets discharged through the vagina as menstrual flow.

About 50 ml of blood will be lost, of which 75% is the arterial and the rest venous. This blood does not clot outside the body as the clotting and fibrinolysis both will have taken place in the uterus itself. *Appearance of clots in the menstrual blood indicates heavy bleeding.*

Hormonal basis of menstrual cycle is as indicated in Fig. 10.5. Upto 10th day and also after the ovulation, usually there is negative feedback over gonadotropin secretion. After 10th day there will be a positive feedback operating which is responsible for LH surge that is essential for ovulation.

Indicators of ovulation

- **Determining basal body temperature** — which is increased by about 0.5 degree Celsius around the day of ovulation and continues throughout the secretory phase. It is due to the thermogenic action of the hormone progesterone.

- **Examination of cervical mucus**—unlike the endometrium of uterus, the cell lining of cervix is not sloughed during bleeding. After ovulation the cervical mucus becomes thick.

- **Endometrial biopsy**.

- Estimation of hormonal levels in circulation.

- Ultra sound examination of follicle.

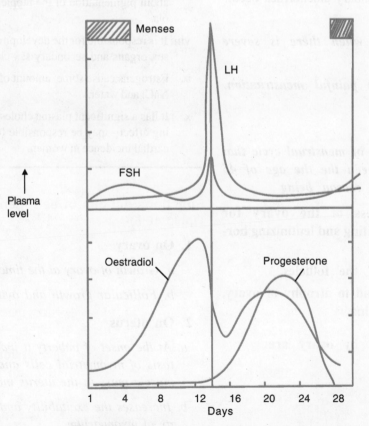

Fig. 10.5 Hormonal levels during a menstrual cycle

Vaginal changes during the menstrual cycle

Under the influence of estrogen the epithelial cell lining of the vagina gets cornified whereas due to the influence of progesterone it will be infiltrated with leucocytes.

Amenorrhea

Absence of menstrual bleeding is known as amenorrhea. There are two types namely primary and secondary amenorrhea. Primary is where menstrual cycles have not started at all. Secondary is when there used to be menstrual cycle but have stopped for some time in between. One of the classical examples where secondary amenorrhea occurs is in pregnancy.

Menorrhagia is when there is severe bleeding.

Dysmenorrhea is painful menstruation.

Menopause

Permanent stoppage of menstrual cycle that usually occurs between the the age of 45 and 50 years. The reason being

- **Non-responsiveness of the ovary for follicular stimulating and leutinizing hormones.**
- **Disappearance of the follicles.**
  The above will lead to atrophy of ovary, uterus and vagina.

Hormones secreted by ovary are

1. *Estrogen*
2. *Progesterone*
3. *Inhibin*
4. *Relaxin.*

Table 10.5 Actions of oestrogen

i.   Facilitates the growth of graffian follicles.

ii. Increase the motility of the uterine tubes.

iii. Is responsible for bringing about changes in the endometrium during the proliferative phase of the menstrual cycle

iv. Increase the amount of muscle mass of the uterus. The uterine muscle becomes more active and more excitable. The uterine muscle becomes more sensitive to oxytocin.

v.   On pituitary glands estrogen decreases FSH and LH secretion most of the times.

vi. Effect on breast - it brings about the enlargement of the breast during puberty and pregnancy. This is due to its action on the duct system. It deposits fat in the breast. It brings about pigmentation of the nipple and the areola.

viii. It is responsible for the development of female sex organs and secondary sex characters.

ix. Estrogens cause some amount of retention of NaCl and water.

x.   It has a significant plasma cholesterol lowering effect - may be responsible for low myocardial incidence in women.

Functions/Actions of estrogen
(Table 10.5)

1. **On ovary**

   a. *Growth of ovary at the time of puberty.*

   b. *Follicular growth and ovulation.*

2. **On uterus**

   a. *At the onset of puberty it induces mitosis of myometrial cells and hence the muscle mass in the uterus increases.*

   b. *Increases the excitability and contractility of myometrium.*

c. In pregnancy, uterus grows to greater extent probably because of increase in muscle length. It also increases the actin and myosin content of muscles.

d. Increases the number of oxytocin receptors.

e. Brings about all the changes in the endometrium during the proliferative phase .

3. On cervix – *secretion will be thin and alkaline. This facilitates the viability and movement of sperms in the female genital tract.*

4. On mammary gland

a. At onset of puberty brings about the development of duct system and branching.

b. Is responsible for deposition of fats.

c. *Is also responsible for pigmentation of areola and nipple.*

5. On skeletal growth

a. *It increases osteoblastic activity and collagen matrix. So facilitates linear growth of body.*

b. Also causes early fusion of epiphyseal plates.

c. *Responsible for narrow shoulder and broad hip development..*

6. On CNS

Makes female more docile and the maternal instincts are due to estrogen hormone.

7. On skin

a. Makes skin smooth, soft and warm.

b. Brings about female type of hair distribution.

8. On redistribution of fats

a. Increases the deposition of fats in hips, breast and thigh.

b. Decreases the cholesterol level. Because of this women before menopause are less prone to myocardial infarction.

Actions of progesterone (Table 10.6)

Table 10.6 Actions of progesterone
i. On the uterus - it is responsible for bringing about progestational (secretory) changes in the uterine endometrium.
ii. It decreases the excitability of the myometrium and makes it less sensitive to the action of oxytocin.
iii. In the breast it brings about the growth and development of the alveoli.
iv. Progesterone has a thermogenic action, responsible for increasing the basal body temperature at the time of ovulation.

1. On uterus

a. Decreases excitability of myometrium and decreases the sensitivity for action of oxytocin.

b. Increases the secretion from the glands of endometrium. It also brings about the coiling of arteries and glands.

2. On mammary glands *causes development of alveoli, which are responsible for secretion of milk.*

3. Responsible for thermogenic actions.

4. Along with estrogen helps in the feed back regulation of secretion **of follicular stimulating and leutinising hormones from the anterior pituitary glands** (Fig. 10.6).

5. Also responsible for thick and acidic secretions of the cervical region.

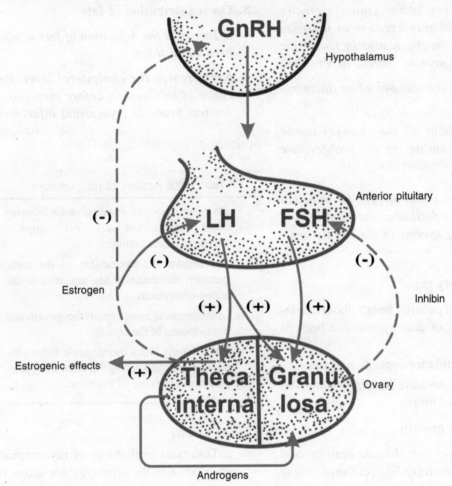

Figure 10.6 Regulation of secretion of ovarian hormones (estrogen and progesterone)

Throughout the menstrual cycle period the free form of estrogen in plasma exerts a negative feedback control over the secretion of FSH and LH from the anterior pituitary glands by acting directly on pituitary as well as through hypothalamus. For the hormonal secretions of the gonads to occur, the hypothalamus should secrete gonadotropin releasing hormone(GnRH). This hormone reaches anterior pituitary gland through the hypothalamo hypophyseal portal system. When this hormone acts on the anterior pituitary gland there will be secretion of FSH and LH. Both these hormones

act on gonads and female sex hormones (estrogen and progesterone) are secreted. During the follicular phase the theca interna cells secrete estrogen and during luteal phase both estrogen and progesterone hormones are secreted by the corpus luteum.

It has to be very much emphasized here that around the day of ovulation when the estrogen level in circulation exceeds a critical value and estrogen instead of exerting a negative feedback control on gonadotropin secretion, now exerts a positive feedback influence. Because of this the LH and FSH levels show a steep rise and sudden fall. Of the two, it is the LH level which increases enormously. This steep rise and fall of LH with a peak, is known as LH surge. This surge is very much essential for the ovulation to be brought about.

HUMAN CHORIONIC GONADOTROPIN (HCG)

1. Another gonadotropic hormone in female is human chorionic gonadotropin.

2. The syncytiotrophoblast cells of placenta secrete this hormone.

3. Since placenta is developed only during pregnancy, HCG secretion occurs during pregnancy.

4. Secretion starts from around 10 days after fertilization.

5. Can be detected in the urine after 4 weeks of last menstruation or in about 2 weeks after fertilization of the ovum.

6. Reaches a peak around 12th week of gestation.

Functions of HCG

1.*Helps for maintenance of corpus luteum and hence prevents involution of corpus luteum. So the hormonal secretions can continue from the corpus luteum till the placenta can take over completely the secretion of oestrogen and progesterone.*

2. *In male fetus it causes the secretion of testosterone from testis and help in descent of testis.*

Immunological test for pregnancy diagnosis

It is based on the presence or absence of human chorionic gonadotropin in the urine *of* the female in question.

Procedure of the test

- *Take a sample of urine of the female.*
- *Add HCG antibodies to it and mix.*
- *After mixing, wait for a minute.*
- *Now add latex particles coated with HCG.*
- **Look for the agglutination of latex particles.**

Observation	Conclusion
No agglutination	the female is <u>PREGNANT</u>.
Agglutination	the female is <u>NOT</u> pregnant

Reason for the conclusion

a. If the female is pregnant, urine contains HCG.

b. When anti HCG antibodies are added, the HCG in the urine neutralizes the anti HCG antibodies.

c. So when the latex particles are added there will be no free antibodies to react with them.

d. Hence there will not be any agglutination.

FUNCTIONS OF PLACENTA

It acts as a bridge as well as a barrier between mother and developing fetus. It has a number of functions. Some of the functions of placenta are

1. **Endocrine function** It secretes a number of hormones. Some of the important hormones secreted are estrogen, progesterone, human chorionic somatotropin, HCG and these hormones have vital role to play during pregnancy.

2. Respiratory function helps for the exchange of gases between fetal and maternal circulations. Oxygen required by the fetus is diffused from the maternal circulation and carbon dioxide diffuses from fetal to maternal circulation.

3. Excretory function: The metabolic waste substances produced in the fetal body can't get excreted directly. Hence these substances are passed on from fetus to maternal circulation for excretion.

4. Nutritive function helps in the diffusion of all vital substances from the maternal to fetal circulation. These substances are needed for the growth and development of fetus.

5. Protective function is because some of the antibodies from maternal circulation can get passed through the placenta to reach fetal body. At the same time some of the antibodies may not get passed through as well (ABO antibodies).

CONTRACEPTION OR FAMILY PLANNING

There are different methods in female and male for avoiding conception. Many of these methods are temporary. But there are permanent methods of contraception as well in male and female.

Contraceptive methods in men

1. Condom *acts as a barrier for deposition of semen into the female genital tract and hence prevents fertilization. But the success rate is only 50%.*

2. Vasectomy *is cutting and ligating of vas deferens.* It is the permanent method of family planning (contraception) in male and is done bi-

laterally. *After vasectomy ejaculation of semen still occurs as 90% of semen is due to secretions from seminal vesicle and prostate gland.* So the volume of semen does not get affected much but sperms will be absent in semen. The person becomes infertile. *After vasectomy the person has to be careful for the next two months or so, as the sperms that have got stored already in the ampulla of vas can still get ejaculated along with semen and lead to conception.*

Contraceptive methods in female

Mechanical methods like use of

1. *Diaphragm, cervical cap.*

2. Intra uterine contraceptive devises (IUD or IUCD) – *devises inserted into the uterus, the most common is copper T.*

   Chemical method **like** *application of spermicides in the form of jelly or tablet into the vagina.*

Hormonal methods

Classical pills that contain estrogen and progesterone. It has to be taken for 21 days, that is from the 5th day of the cycle to 25th day. The probable mechanism of action of the pills is

a. Prevents LH surge due to constant negative feedback influence and hence prevents ovulation

b. The progesterone present in the tablet makes the endocervical secretions thick and acidic. So the viability of sperms is affected and also the motility of sperms. Hence there may not be fertilization even if there is ovulation

c. *Makes the endometrium hostile and prevents implantation of the zygote.*

Tubectomy

Is the only permanent method of family planning in female. In this method there will be bilateral cutting and ligating of fallopian tubes. When this is done the continuity of the fallopian is lost and hence there is no chance for the sperms to come across with the ovum. Because of this there will not be any fertilization.

Other methods of contraception, which can't be categorized as specifically in male or female, are

- Rhythm method (safe period)
- Coitus interruptus

Rhythm method (safe period)

a. *It is based on the presumption of number of days in a cycle.*

b. *But there are chances that the number of days of each cycle may vary in the same individual.*

c. *Hence it is not a very successful method.*

Assuming that the cycle duration of 28 days, the following need to be explained:

1. *In a 28 day cycle the ovulation normally occurs around 14th day. It can also occur one or two days on either side.*

2. The sperms are viable in the female genital tract for about 24-72 hours.

3. *The ovum is viable in the female genital tract for about 24-48 hours.*

Because of the aforesaid reasons it is safe to have sexual intercourse from day 5 to day 9 and from day 20 to day 28 in a 28 day cycle. If there is sexual intercourse between day 10 and day 19 it is a very high risk or unsafe period.

Coitus interruptus

In this method, just before ejaculation, the penis is withdrwan from the vagina. so the deposition of semen into the vagina is prevented. this is not a very safe method of family planning.

Questions

All major questions are of 8-10 marks.

All short note type questions 4 marks each.

CARDIOVASCULAR SYSTEM

Major questions

1. Give the normal values of blood pressure. Explain the reflex regulation of arterial blood pressure.

2. Describe how blood pressure is regulated after blood loss.

3. Explain the function of arterial baroreceptors in the regulation of blood pressure.

4. What are baroreceptors? Mention their locations. Describe their role in regulation of blood pressure.

5. Define blood pressue. Describe the baroreceptors and hormones in the regulation of blood pressure.

6. Describe the factors determining cardiac output.

7. Define cardiac output and cardiac index. Describe the regulation of cardiac output.

8. Using pressure tracings describe the events that occur on the left side of heart during a cardiac cycle.

9. Draw diagram to show the relation between left intraventricular pressure and aortic pressure. Describe the events during ventricular cycle.

10. Define circulatory shock. Give the physiological basis for the features of hypovolemic shock.

Short notes

1. With the help of composite diagram, describe the pressure and volume changes in right ventricle during a cardiac cycle.

2. What is phonocardiogram? Tabulate the differences between first and second heart sounds.

3. List four uses of ECG. Explain any one.

4. Draw a normal ECG recorded from limb lead II. Give the cause for different waves.

5. What is P-R interval? How is measured? What is its significance?

6. Briefly outline four uses of ECG in clinical practice.

7. Describe the factors, which regulate cardiac output.

8. How much is end diastolic volume? Explain the mechanism of ventricular filling.

9. Explain Frank Starling's law of heart and its application.

10. List factors influencing venous return. Explain any one.

11. Explain triple response.

12. Explain the salient features of cerebral blood flow.

13. Give Poiseuille Hagen formula. Based on this, briefly explain the factors regulating blood flow to an organ.

14. Give normal value of coronary blood flow. Explain how coronary blood flow is regulated.

15. Define peripheral resistance. Explain its basis, regulation and significance.

16. Define peripheral resistance. Enumerate the factors that alter it. Explain how it affects blood pressure.

17. Enumerate any four properties of cardiac muscle. Explain any two.

18. Briefly explain any two special properties of cardiac muscle.

19. Explain Frank Starling's law of heart.

20. What is cardiac catheterization? Mention any two uses.

21. Explain the importance of vagal tone.

22. What is normal heart rate in adult at rest? Explain the factors that regulate heart rate.

23. Define arteriolar tone and veno motor tone. Briefly explain how are they maintained.

24. Define systolic, diastolic, pulse and mean arterial pressures and give the normal values.

25. Briefly explain CNS ischemic response in the regulation of blood pressure.

BLOOD

Major questions

1. Explain the changes occurring in the erythroid precursors during erythropoiesis. Name any four hemopoietic factors. Explain the mechanism of any one.

2. Describe the changes that occur in erythropoiesis. With the help of the flow chart describe the regulation of red blood cell count.

3. Describe formation, transport and excretion of bilirubin. Explain the changes in urine in post hepatic jaundice.

4. Name the blood group systems. Explain the importance of blood groups. Explain the precaution to be taken before and during blood transfusion.

5. What is Landsteiner's law? Explain its application in ABO and Rh system. Describe in detail the complications of mismatched transfusion.

6 Outline the principle and procedure for determining blood group of an individual. Explain the significance of Rh system.

7. Describe the morphology and functions of white blood cells.

8. What is the basis for classification of leucocytes. With the help of labeled diagrams, describe the morphology of each type of cell.

9. Describe the functions of plasma albumin and globulins. Give the causes and consequences of low plasma albumin level.

10. Draw a schematic diagram to show the intrinsic pathway of blood coagulation. Name any four anticoagulants and explain the mechanism of action of each.

11. Give a schematic diagram and explain process of blood coagulation in a test tube. Explain how intra vascular clotting is prevented.

12. Describe the natural mechanisms responsible for arrest of bleeding from small blood vessels.

Short type questions

1. Name blood group systems. Explain the importance of blood groups.

2. Describe the complications of mismatched blood transfusion.

3. In a tabular column indicate the agglutinogen and agglutinin present in ABO system of blood grouping.

4. What is erythroblastosis fetalis? Give its basis and principle of treatment.

5. Define anticoagulants. Name any four and give the mechanism of action of any one.

6. How are anticoagulants classified? Name any two and give the mechanism of action of each.

7. Explain the mechanism of action of heparin and dicoumarol.

8. How is clotting normally prevented inside the blood vessels.

9. Write briefly one the fibrinolytic mechanism. Name any one drug which can be used in thrombolysis.

10. Outline the extrinsic pathway of blood coagulation. Add a note on prothrombin time.

11. Write briefly on the functions of platelets.

12. Explain how vitamin K deficiency is associated with coagulation disorder.

13. Write briefly on cause and features of themophilia.

14. What is edema? Name any two common causes for the same. Explain the mechanism of development of edema in any one cause.

15. Give an account of clotting disorders.

16. What is anemia? Enumerate the various types of anemia and explain how any two types are caused.

17. Define and state the significance of i. Hematocrit ii. Erythrocyte sedimentation rate.

18. Name the erythropoietic factors. Explain the effects on red cells when any two are deficient.

19. Explain the steps in phagocytosis.

20. Outline the role of lymphocytes in immunity.

21. Briefly explain the functions of lymphocytes.

22. Distinguish between the function of T and B lymphocytes.

23. Explain the role of neutrophil in defense function.

24. Give the composition of blood. Write briefly on any three functions.

25. How is lymph formed? Explain how edema occurs in lymph vessel blockade.

GI TRACT
SALIVA AND DEGLUTITION

Minor Questions:

1. Explain 'reflex salivation'.

2. Explain how salivary secretion is brought about: i) when food is placed in the mouth. ii) at the though of food.

3. Name the important constituents of saliva and explain the functions of any three **components.**

4. Explain the reflex effects produced during deglutition.

5. Describe the events in 2nd phase of deglutition.

6. Describe the oesophageal phase of deglutition. What is achalacia cardia?

GASTRIC

Major Questions

1. Describe the regulation of secretion of gastric juice in different phases of secretion.

2. Enumerate four functions of stomach and explain any one. Describe how gastric secretion is studied experimentally.

3. Give the pH, constituents and functions of gastric juice. Describe the cephalic phase of gastric juice secretion.

Minor Questions

4. Explain the regulation of cephalic phase of gastric secretion .

5. Outline the regulation of gastric phase of gastric secretion.

6. Name the different types of cells in the gastric mucosa and specify the function of each.

7. Explain the factors which influence gastric motility and emptying.

8. Explain the physiological basis of treatment of peptic ulcer.

9. List four important components of gastric juice. Explain functions of any one component.

PANCREAS AND SMALL INTESTINE

Minor Questions

1. List the functions and regulations of secretion of pancreatic secretion.

2. Enumerate the constituents of pancreatic juice. Describe the regulation of pancreatic juice.

3. Give the pH and important constituents pancreatic juice. Describe how it is regulated.

BILE, LIVER AND DIGESTION

Major Questions

1. Describe functions of bile. Add a note on regulation of bile secretion and release.

2. Describe the secretion, storage and release of bile. Explain the functions of bile salts.

3. Describe the role of bile in digestion and absorption of fats.

Minor Questions

4. Give two differences between hepatic bile and gall bladder bile and account for these differences. Explain the effects of removal of gall bladder.

5. Name the bile salts and describe their functions.

6. Enumerate four functions of liver. Explain two liver function tests.

LARGE INTESTINE

Minor Questions

1. Explain the 'defecation reflex'.

2. Explain the functions of colon.

MOVEMENTS

Minor Questions

1. Outline the mechanism of peristalsis.

2. Explain the role of different types of small intestinal movements.

3. Name the different intestinal movements. Explain the role of any one.

MISCELLANEOUS

Major and Minor Questions

1. List four gastrointestinal hormones. Describe the actions of nay three hormones.

2. Name two major gastrointestinal hormones and describe actions of any one hormone.

3. Outline the actions of any two gastrointestinal hormones.

RENAL, SKIN AND TEMPERATURE REGULATION

Major Questions

1. Name the basic steps in the formation of urine. Explain the changes brought about by the renal tubules on fluid from the Bowman's capsule.

2. Describe the reabsorption of water and sodium in the renal tubular.

Minor Questions

3. Describe the micturition reflex. In adults, give i) volume at which sense of fullness is first felt ii) volume at which there is a sense of urgency to void.

4. Give the normal value of renal blood flow (RBF). Explain the principle of Renal Plasma Flow.

5. Explain briefly the importance of countercurrent multiplier system in renal function.

6. Explain the functions of distal convoluted tubule and collecting duct of nephron.

7. Explain the terms "Transport maximum" and 'renal threshold' using glucose as an example. Give three normal values for glucose.

8. What are vasarecta? Briefly explain their role in renal function.

9. Explain glucose reabsorption in the nephron.

10. Define micturition. Draw micturition reflex arc.

11. Draw and describe cystometrogram.

12. Draw a diagram to show the components of juxta glomerular apparatus. Enumerate the functions of juxta glomerular apparatus.

13. Describe the effects of ADH on renal tubules and its effects on urine formation.

14. Give a short account of the function of renal tubules.

15. Define renal threshold for glucose. Explain the effect produced when the plasma glucose exceeds renal threshold.

16. Explain the differences between water reabsorption in proximal convoluted tubule and collecting duct.

17. Describe tubular reabsorption of glucose.

18. Enumerate the factors affecting the glomerular filtration pressure and explain their role.

19. Explain how water and sodium are handled by proximal convoluted tubules of kidney.

20. Describe briefly water reabsorption in the renal tubules.

21. Give a brief account of the mechanism(s) by which heat is lost from the body.

22. Give the location of thermoreceptors. Explain the role of skin in the regulation of body temperature.

23. Outline the role of the skin in body temperature regulation in a cold environment.

24. Describe the role of skin in temperature regulation.

25. Enumerate the functions of skin in temperature regulation. Explain any one.

26. Where are the temperature regulating centers located? Explain the mechanisms by which body heat is conserved.

27. Define glomerular filtration rate (GFR). Explain how is it regulated.

28. Define the term "renal clearance". Explain significance of insulin clearance.

29. Define micturition. With the help of a diagram describe micturition reflex.

30. Describe the factors which favour and oppose glomerular filtration.

RESPIRATION
VENTILATION

Minor Questions

1. Define intrapleural pressure. How is it caused? Explain how it varies during the respiratory cycle.

2. Explain the role of surfactant in pulmonary function.

3. Outline the mechanism of quiet inspiration and expiration.

4. What is timed vital capacity? Give its importance as a lung function test.

5. What is pulmonary surfactant? Describe the effects of lack of surfactant in lungs.

6. Explain how negative intra alveolar pressure is achieved. Mention its effects.

7. Define vital capacity. Name two other tests of ventilatory function and give the significance of each.

TRANSPORT

Minor Questions

1. Describe the role of Haldane effect in the transport of CO_2.

2. Explain the factors governing gas exchange at lungs.

3. Explain the advantages of thee shape of oxygen dissociation curve of hemoglobin. Enumerate factors shifting the curve to the right.

4. Name the forms in which CO_2 is transported in the blood. Explain Haldane effect.

REGULATION

Major Questions

1. Mention the location of respiratory chemoreceptors. Describe their role in the regulation of respiration.

2. Name the locations of the respiratory centers. Explain their role in bringing about normal rhythmic respiration. Mention the effects of acute asphyxia on respiration.

3. Give a brief account of chemical regulation of respiration.

Minor Questions

4. Give the location of respiratory chemoreceptors. Explain the role of these receptors in the regulation of respiration.

5. Explain the effects on respiration of acclimatization to high altitude. Mention the purpose of these effects.

MISCELLANEOUS

Minor Questions

1. Explain the basis of symptoms of decompression sickness. Mention how it can be prevented.

2. Define dyspnoea and apnoea. Give two examples each when dyspnoea and apnoea occur.

3. Define cyanosis. Explain its development and significance.

4. Name the different types of hypoxias. Mention in which type(s) of hypoxia, cyanosis is seen and explain the reason for its occurrence.

5. a) Explain the functions of the nose.

   b) List the nonchemical influences to the respiratory centers and explain the role of any

6. Explain the causes and features of hypoxia. Add a note on mountain sickness.

CENTRAL NERVOUS SYSTEM
SYNAPSE, REFLEXES, RECEPTORS AND SENSATIONS

Major Questions

1. Give any <u>one</u> classification of sensory receptors with examples. Explain the following aspects of receptor function (a) Adequate stimulus (b) Specificity of receptors (c) Intensity discrimination (d) Adaptation.

2. Draw a diagram to show the pain pathways from limbs. Using this knowledge, four procedures various ways to relieve pain.

3. What is referred pain? Explain its mechanism.

4. Name the Proprioceptors. Draw a diagram to show the pathways which carry impulses from them.

5. Name four ascending tracts of spinal cord. Draw a labeled diagram to show the pathway for fine touch.

Minor Questions

6. Enumerate two properties of a sensory receptor. Explain how receptors are useful in sensory perception.

7. Give the effects of cutting of a series of dorsal nerve roots.

8. Explain the normal plantar reflex. What happens to the plantar reflex in: i) Lesion to Pyramidal tract ii) Infants.

9. Define reflex action. What are the components of a reflex arc? Give the clinical significance of reflexes.

10. What is a synapse? Mention the different types of typical synapses. Name any <u>four</u> synaptic transmitters.

11. What is referred pain? Give two examples. Explain its basis.

12. Define reflex action. Draw a diagram of the reflex arc. How do you classify reflexes clinically?

13. What is stereognosis? How is it tested clinically? Name the tract that mediates it.

14. Draw labeled diagrams of pathways of touch sensations from left foot.

15. Explain the terms: i) presynaptic inhibition ii) postsynaptic inhibition with diagrams.

16. What is referred pain? What are the theories regarding referred pain? Give two examples of referred pain.

SPINAL CORD, MOTOR, BASAL GANGLIA, CEREBELLUM

Major Questions

1. Describe the functions of cerebellum. Explain four clinical manifestations of cerebellar lesions.

2. Give the neural connections and functions of Basal Ganglia. Explain the effects of lesions of Nigrostriatal pathway.

3. Name the functional divisions of the cerebellum. Explain four clinical manifestations of cerebellar lesions.

4. Name the sensations carried by dorsal column tracts. Draw a diagram of the pathway for fine touch. Explain dissociated anaesthesia.

5. Explain the changes seen below the level of lesion with a hemisection of the spinal cord at the midthoracic level on the right side give their basis of the change.

6. Describe the immediate effects of complete transection of the spinal cord at midthoracic level. Explain how recovery of reflex activity occurs. Give the probable basis of the changes.

7. Name four ascending tracts. Draw a labeled diagram to show the origin, course and termination f the corticospinal tract. Define hemiplegia. Explain the features of hemiplegia.

8. Name the functional components of the basal ganglia. Describe the features of Parkinsonism. Give their physiological basis.

9. Draw a diagram of the pyramidal tract to show its origin, course and termination. Mention its functions. Explain the features of a lesion to this tract in left internal capsule.

10. Enumerate the salient features of Parkinson's disease. Give the pathway involved and the basis for its treatment.

11. Describe the effects of a lower motor neuron lesion. Name a common disease affecting the lower motor neurons.

12. Enumerate four clinical features of Parkinson's disease. Explain one feature.

13. Enumerate four effects of cerebellar lesions. Explain any two.

VESTIBULAR APPARATUS

1. Describe the otolith organs and their functions.

CORTEX AND CSF

Minor Questions

1. Outline the formation, circulation and functions of cerebrospinal fluid.

2. What is cerebrospinal fluid (CSF)? Name the sites of formation, circulation and drainage and functions of CSF. Add a note on lumbar puncture.

3. Explain three functions of cerebrospinal fluid. How is a sample of CSF obtained?

HYPOTHALAMUS, THALAMUS, RETICULAR FORMATION, ECG, SLEEP

Major Questions

1. Describe any four functions of hypothalamus with relevant connections. Add a note on 'Hypothalamic obesity'.

2. Describe the hypothalamic regulation of food intake.

Minor Questions

3. List four functions of hypothalamus. Explain <u>one</u> of them.

4. What is EEG? What are its normal waves? What is alpha block?

5. What is electroencephalography? Describe its various waves.

6. Enumerate the functions of reticular formation. Explain any one.

7. Give an account of the connections and functions of the thalamus. Explain the cause of thalamic syndrome and name two features.

8. List four functions of reticular formation. Explain any two.

9. Enumerate four functions of the hypothalamus. Describe any two functions. Explain two features of hypothalamus disorders.

REPRODUCTION
MALE

Minor Questions

1. Explain how growth, development and functioning of sexual organs is regulated by testosterone.

2. Explain the effect of castration before puberty and after puberty.

3. Describe the endocrine functions of testis.

4. What are the effects of castration in male a) before puberty and b) after puberty.

FEMALE

Major Questions

1. Describe the normal ovarian cycle and its regulation.

Minor Questions

2. List four indicators of ovulation. Explain the basis of a method that can be done in an out patient clinic.

3. Describe the changes in the endometrium during menstrual cycle. Specify the hormones responsible for each phase.

4. When does ovulation occur in a 30 day menstrual cycle? Mention the hormones responsible for ovulation.

5. Enumerate the functions of the placenta. Explain any one.

6. Explain any two methods for determining ovulation. Give their physiological basis.

7. List four methods of contraception in the female. Explain the Physiological basis of any one of them.

8. List four functions of the placenta. Explain any <u>one</u> of them.

9. When does ovulation occur in a menstrual cycle with a duration of 32 days. Name tow indicators of ovulation. Explain any two tests of ovulation.

10. What are oral contraceptives? Explain the physiological basis of oral contraceptive pills.

11. Define ovulation. List two reliable tests of ovulation and give their physiological basis.

12. Explain the role of oxytocin in bringing about delivery of the foetus.

13. Describe: a) Formation and role of corpus luteum b) Functions of Sertoli cells.

14. Explain the functions of a) Corpus luteum b) Sertoli cells.

ENDOCRINE
ANTERIOR AND POSTERIOR PITUITARY

Major Questions

1. Describe physiological actions and control of secretion of growth hormone. Explain the consequences of its hyper-and hyposecretion <u>before puberty</u>.

2. Enumerate the hormones of the anterior pituitary gland. Describe the regulation of secretion of any <u>one</u> of them.

3. Explain how a pituitary dwarf if different from a cretin.

4. Explain the actions and regulation of secretion of any one hormones of posterior pituitary gland.

5. Explain with the help of a labeled diagram the hypothalamic control of the posterior pituitary. Describe the functions and regulation of secretion of oxytocin.

Minor Questions

6. Explain the features and basis of i) Gigantism ii) Acromegaly.

7. Draw a diagram to show how secretion of ACTH is regulated. What are its actions?

8. Explain role of ADH in relating water balance in the body.

9. Outline the role of Antidiuretic hormone.

10. Name the hormones of the neurohypophysis. Describe their actions.

11. Define/explain neuroendocrine reflex. Describe the role of any two neuro endocrine reflexes.

12. Explain three features of diabetes insipidus.

THYROID

Major Questions

1. Outline the steps in the synthesis of thyroid hormones. Explain the role of thyroid hormones in growth and development.

2. Describe the synthesis, release and functions of thyroid hormones.

Minor Questions

3. Name four features of Cretinism. Explain their basis.

4. List four features of hypothyroidism in a child. Explain the basis of any two features.

5. Name two features of hyperthyroidism. Explain the basis of each feature.

6. Explain the effects of thyroid hormones on development and functioning of nervous system.

7. Draw a diagram to show the taste pathway from the anterior 2/3 of the tongue. Explain the meaning of the terms "ageusia and dysgeusia".

8. Explain the role of the chemical senses.

9. Name the primary taste sensations. Draw a diagram of taste pathway.

PARATHYROID

Major Questions

1. Specify the influence of parathormone, calcitonin and 1-25(OH2) calciferol on blood calcium concentration. Explain the mechanism of action of any one of them.

2. Describe the role of hormones in calcium homeostasis.

3. List the functions of calcium in the body. Describe calcium homeostasis.

Minor Questions

4. What is tetany? Explain its clinical features.

5. Explain the role of parathormone.

BLOOD SUGAR

Major Questions

1. Give the source and physiological effects of a hypoglycemic hormone. Mention the consequences of its deficiency.

2. List four differences between diabetes insipidus and diabetes mellitus.

Minor Questions

3. Explain the hypoglycemic actions of insulin.

<hr>

ADRENAL

Major Questions

1. Discuss the source, physiological actions and regulation of secretion a mineralo corticoid.

2. Name the glucocorticoids and their source. Describe the physiological actions of glucocorticoids

3. List four characteristic features of Cushing's syndrome. Explain the basis for each of these features.

4. Give an account of the various physiological actions of glucocorticoids.

5. Describe the action of glucocorticoids on the following: a) blood cells b) inflammation and allerty c) carbohydrate metabolism d) water and electrolyte metabolism.

Minor Questions

6. Explain four changes seen in Cushing's syndrome.

7. Describe briefly the factors regulating the secretion of mineralocorticoids.

8. Name the hormones secreted by the adrenal medulla. Compare their actions on CVS. Classify the adrenergic receptors and name one blocker for each type of receptor.

<hr>

GENERAL

Major Questions

1. Explain the different mechanisms by which the secretion of hormones is regulated, giving one example for each.

Minor Questions

2. Classify hormones based on their chemical nature. Explain the mechanisms by which they act.

3. Explain permissive action of hormones giving examples.

<hr>

SPECIAL SENSES
EYE

Minor Questions

1. What is colour blindness? What are its different types? Explain two methods to test colour vision.

2. Describe the phenomenon of dark adaptation in the eye.

3. Describe the functions of iris.

4. Draw diagrams to show image formation in prebyopia. Give its basis and correction.

5. What is field of vision? Indicate on a diagram, the field defect when there is a lesion of the left optic tract.

6. Enumerate the functions of the retinal receptors.

7. Draw a diagram of the visual pathway. Describe the effects of pressure on the optic chiasma.

8. Describe the papillary reflexes. What is means by the Argyll Robertson pupil?

9. What is dark adaptation? Explain how it occurs. Name one condition in which dark adaptation is prolonged.

10. Mention the changes occurring in accommodation for near vision. Explain the purpose of each change.

11. Compare the functions of the retinal receptors.

12. Explain the terms, far point and near point vision. Explain why the near point of vision recedes throughout life.

13. Name the primary colours. Describe the Young-Helmholtz theory of colour vision.

HEARING

Minor Questions

1. Explain the "traveling wave" theory of hearing.

2. List four functions of the middle ear. Explain any one.

3. Draw a labeled diagram of the auditory pathway. Give two special features of its pathway.

4. How is hearing affected in a lesion of i) left cochlear nerve ii) right temporal lobe. Give reasons for your answers.

5. Name the contents of the middle ear and explain their functions.

6. Explain the role of the middle ear in hearing.

MUSCLE

Minor Questions

1. Explain any four differences in the functional properties of skeletal muscle and smooth muscle.

2. In a tabular statement give any four differences in the functional properties of skeletal muscle and smooth muscle.

3. Give the components and functions of the sarcotubular system in skeletal muscle. How does it differ from cardiac muscle?

4. Define motor unit. Describe its relation to muscle contraction.

5. Define refractory period. Explain its basis and significance.

6. Draw a labeled diagram of a sarcomere and indicate the different bands. Explain the role of sarcoplasmic triad.

7. What is motor unit? Give its physiological importance.

8. Draw and define a motor unit. What is quantal summation?

NERVE

Minor Questions

1. Draw diagrams to show how nerve impulse is propagated in a (i) myelinated nerve (ii) Non-myelinated nerve.

2. Give in a table the types of nerve fibers, their diameters, conduction rates and functions.

3. Explain the basis for the resting membrane potential of a nerve fibre.

4. Draw a monophasic nerve action potential. Explain how it differs from a compound action potential.

5. Explain the process of nerve regeneration after a peripheral nerve is cut. List two important factors that affect regeneration.

6. Explain the ionic basis of resting membrane potential of a nerve fibre.

7. Define chronaxie and rheobase. Draw a diagram of the strength duration curve and mark therein rheobase and chronaxie. Give the significance of chronaxie.

8. Draw a monophasic action potential. Specify the ionic basis of the various phases.

NEUROMUSCULAR JUNCTION

Minor Questions

1. Classify neuromuscular blockers. Explain the mechanism of action of any two.

2. List the sequence of events which causes transmission of impulse across neuromuscular junction.

3. Enumerate the steps by which a motor nerve impulse leads to connection of skeletal muscle.

4. List the steps in neuromuscular transmission in skeletal muscle. Give the basis of myasthenia gravis.

5. Name two neuromuscular blocking drugs. Explain the mechanism(s) of action of each. Mention two uses of these drugs.

Index